Atlas of
NASAL CYTOLOGY
for the Differential Diagnosis
of Nasal Diseases

Matteo Gelardi

Atlas of
NASAL CYTOLOGY
for the Differential Diagnosis
of Nasal Diseases

English translation revision by John F. Pallanch, M.D., M.S., F.A.C.S.

Division Chair of Rhinology
Mayo Clinic
Rochester, Minnesota (USA)

Second edition

edi·ermes

ATLAS of NASAL CYTOLOGY for the Differential Diagnosis of Nasal Diseases
by Matteo Gelardi
SECOND EDITION

Copyright 2012 Edi.Ermes - New York (USA)

ISBN 978-1-4675-3035-4

Copyright 2012 Edi.Ermes - Milan (Italy) - Italian edition ISBN 978-88-7051-372-1

A book is the end product of a very complex series of operations that include numerous checks, of both the text and the images. It is almost impossible to publish a volume entirely free of errors. We would therefore be very grateful to be notified of any found in this book.
For any remarks or suggestions about this book, please contact us at the following address:
External Relations - Edi.Ermes srl - Viale Enrico Forlanini, 65 - 20134 Milan, Italy
e-mail: international@eenet.eu

Drawings: Andrea Rossi Raccagni/the Edi.Ermes archive

English translation revision: Catherine Wrenn (Italy)

Printed in April 2012 by Arti Grafiche Colombo - Gessate (MI) - Italy
for Edi.Ermes - viale Enrico Forlanini, 65 - 20134 Milan, Italy
http://www.ediermes.it - Tel. ++39 02.70.21.121 - Fax ++39 02.70.21.12.83

FOREWORD

Atlas of Nasal Cytology for the Differential Diagnosis of Nasal Diseases is a landmark work by the world's foremost expert on nasal cytology, Matteo Gelardi.

Unlike the lungs and ears, the nose is a part of the respiratory tract from which it is possible to readily obtain a sample of the cells that represent the current status of the health or disease of the tissue and mucous. Because of the dedicated work of Matteo Gelardi over the past 20 years, a growing number of physicians now take advantage of the unique and valuable information that is available for the diagnosis of nasal conditions by studying samples of the cells from the nose. This second edition is particularly valuable as an update for them, as well as for any physician who cares for patients with nasal disorders.

The second edition adds outstanding illustrations and additional areas of coverage to the already invaluable first edition. The coverage of additional subject matter enhances an already valuable book in augmenting the practitioner's ability to diagnose and optimally treat conditions of the nose.

The reader will find that a new world is opened to them as they study this text. Rhinologic diagnosis will ultimately be universally refined by these techniques. Those who wish to be on the cutting edges of diagnosis and optimal treatment in Rhinology will find this book to be a critical tool in their armamentarium.

John Pallanch, M.D., M.S., F.A.C.S.
Division Chair of Rhinology
Mayo Clinic
Rochester, Minnesota (USA)

PREFACE TO THE SECOND EDITION

Over the past 20 years, advances in technology and scientific research have radically changed the clinical approach to diagnosis and treatment. In rhinology, for example, besides history taking, numerous diagnostic procedures (rhinomanometry, acoustic rhinometry, endoscopy, immunohistochemistry, immunologic tests) facilitate diagnosis and treatment planning.

Nasal cytology is an additional diagnostic method. Yet despite its simplicity and proven utility in giving direction to the diagnostic study of many nasal diseases such as allergic rhinitis, NARES (non allergic rhinitis with eosinophilia syndrome), NARNE (non allergic rhinitis with neutrophils), NARMA (non allergic rhinitis with mast cells) and, among the most recent discoveries, the new nosological entity called NARESMA (non allergic rhinitis with eosinophils and mast cells), nasal cytology paradoxically remains underused. Perhaps this is because nasal cytology is thought to be an unattractive modality by multinational companies that prefer to promote high-tech instruments instead. In fact, the only apparatus required for nasal cytology is a standard light microscope, which costs far less than the instruments required for conducting the more sophisticated studies mentioned above.

But lack of sponsorship is not the only obstacle to a wider use of nasal cytology. A major difficulty anyone wishing to use this method will have noticed is the lack of textbooks and atlases about this discipline, a subject that is not even on the medical school curriculum. Nasal cytology merits greater attention, given that its origins date back to 1889, when Gollash studied the nasal secretions of an asthmatic patient and found numerous eosinophils, leading to the recognition of their role in the pathogenesis of this disorder. Over the years, other researchers reported the importance of nasal cytology (Eyrmann, 1927; Johnson and Goldstein, 1932), but it was not until 1950 with the work of Bryans that nasal cytology started to become better known.

The importance of nasal cytology is based on a fundamental concept. The rhinocytogram of a healthy individual is composed of cells that normally make up the ciliated pseudostratified epithelium: ciliated and non ciliated columnar cells, mucous cells and basal cells. Occasionally neutrophils, and rarely bacteria, can be found. The presence of other cell types such as mast cells, eosinophils, spores or numerous bacteria prompts suspicion of a specific nasal disease.

Nasal cytology can aid in distinguishing inflammatory rhinopathies from infectious nasal diseases, allergic rhinitis from non allergic conditions, and bacterial from viral causes. Moreover, the methodology can also identify mycotic infections, which have come under scrutiny for their possible correlation with the pathogenesis of nasal polyposis. It also makes it possible to diagnose, in a single patient, the simultaneous occurance of more than one rhinopathology (e.g. allergic rhinitis associated with NARES).

Two advantages that make nasal cytology a practical tool affordable to most rhinology-allergy services for clinical diagnosis are:
- its simplicity of use;
- its minimal invasiveness. The procedure does not require anesthesia, thus permitting repeated control examinations as needed.

Equally important is the role nasal cytology plays in scientific research. It allows the evaluation of cell behavior under various conditions. The nasal mucosa is exposed to contact with the external environment, and thus is open to attack from physical, chemical, bacterial and viral agents and other pathogens. Using nasal cytology, the course of a disease can be followed and the response to treatment monitored and evaluated.

This atlas provides the theoretical content and a selection of images from the cytological picture library discussed in the practical sessions of my Masters course in nasal cytology which I have run since 2003. Its 42 sessions have been attended by over 900 specialists from various branches of medicine (otolaryngologists, allergists, pediatricians, pulmonologists and biologists), some of whom have very enthusiastically embraced this fascinating and useful diagnostic approach. This experience resulted in the training of nasal cytology specialists and led to the formation, nationally level, of a special study group. This, in turn, led to the creation of the Italian Academy of Nasal Cytology (Accademia Italiana di Citologia Nasale, AICNA).

Starting in 2011, in the wake of my exciting experience in Italy, I have organized Masters courses in nasal cytology at the international level, accredited by the European Union of Medical Specialists (Union Européenne des Médecins Spécialistes, UEMS), where I encountered, among the participants, great interest in diagnostic nasal cytology.

It is important to recall some of the many scientific contributions made by diagnostic nasal cytology over the past decade. They include not only cytomorphologic insights but, particularly, clinical-diagnostic and therapeutic elements.

In particular, it is worth remembering, in addition to the previously mentioned "NARESMA" and the concept of "overlapping" of more than one rhinopathology (e.g. allergic rhinitis associated with NARES), the identification of "infectious spots" which are morphologic-chromatic expressions of biofilm, clinical-cytological grading and the prognostic index of relapse in nasal polyposis. These achievements give us an incentive to continue our research, with great enthusiasm, and to look for more and more alliances in the scientific field.

The atlas is directed toward respiratory disease specialists working in ORL, allergy, pulmonology and pediatrics who wish to learn the theoretical basis of and correct methodology for modern cytology, as well as the ability to recognize and interpret cellular variations that occur during the course of nasal diseases.

These prerequisite skills represent the essential components of a diagnostic strategy, which, now more than ever, is directed at a more rational, efficacious, and less costly diagnostic-therapeutic program.

To conclude, I wish to express my gratitude to my dear friend John Pallanch, MD, rhinologist, Mayo College of Medicine, Rochester, Minnesota, USA, who kindly accepted the task of editing the English edition of this atlas.

Bari, January 2012

Matteo Gelardi
Head of the Rhinology Unit
Clinic of Otorhinolaryngology
"Policlinico di Bari" University Hospital
University of Bari

to my wife Anna,
my three children,
Genny, Stefania and Giuseppe
and... to my "adoptive" family
the Italian Academy
of Nasal Cytology (AICNA)

SHORT BIOGRAPHY

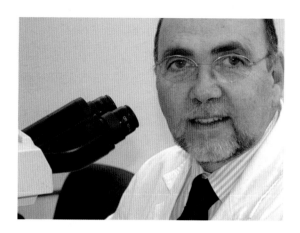

Matteo Gelardi is a specialist in otorhinolaryngology, with specific expertise in clinical allergy and immunology, as well as in morphometric and immunohistochemical techniques applied to clinical oncology.

Within rhinology, Dr Gelardi specializes in nasal cytology. His studies focus on defense mechanisms and cytologic alterations that occur during upper airway infection. This work has earned him wide recognition in Italy and abroad.

Formerly adjunct professor at the Schools of Specialization in Otorhinolaryngology of the Universities of Padua and Ferrara, lecturing in rhinologic symptomatology and nasal cytology, Matteo Gelardi is currently "Head of the Rhinology Unit" at the Clinic of Otorhinolaryngology, "Policlinico di Bari" University Hospital, University of Bari.

His academic duties include his role as invited professor of rhinologic symptomatology and nasal cytology in the postgraduate program for specialization in otorhinolaryngology at the University of Padua and Ferrara.

He was coordinator and instructor in the postgraduate program for specialization in otorhinolaryngology at the University of Bari.

He has published in leading scientific journals (e.g. *Lancet, American Journal of Rhinology, Journal of Allergy and Clinical Immunology, Allergy, British Journal of Sports Medicine*) and has been a speaker at numerous national and international conferences.

He is author of the first "Atlas of Nasal Cytology" (Centro Scientifico Editore, 2004) which was translated into English in 2007.

Particularly active in continuing education in nasal cytology, Dr Gelardi regularly organizes Masters courses accredited by the Ministry of Health for specialists in upper airway infections (otorhinolaryngologists, pediatricians, allergists, pulmonologists, etc.). Since 2011 he has organized, internationally, Masters courses in nasal cytology, accredited by the European Union of Medical Specialists (UEMS).

Since 2008, he has been a member of the Italian Guidelines Commission for the global ARIA (Allergic Rhinitis and its Impact on Asthma) project.

He is a member of the Italian Society of Otorhinolaryngology (SIO) and the Italian Society of Cytology (SICI).

In 2009 he founded, together with his students, the Italian Academy of Nasal Cytology (AICNA), of which he is currently president.

He has also created a website (www.citologianasale.it), containing information about diagnostic cytology.

FIRST MASTER IN NASAL CYTOLOGY COURSE
Bari, November 2002

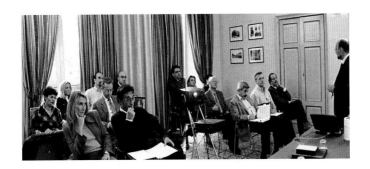

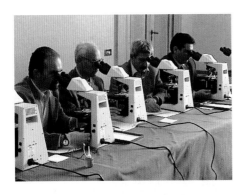

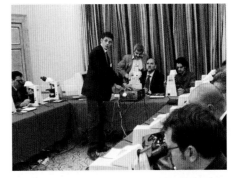

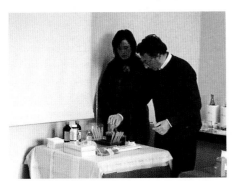

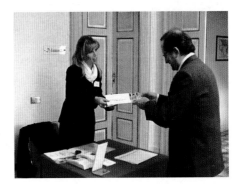

CONTENTS

1. THE CELL 1
    Cell Morphology 2
    The Nucleus 3
        Chromatin 3
        The Nucleoplasm 4
        The Nuclear membrane 4
        The Nucleolus 5
    The Cytoplasm 6
        The Golgi Apparatus 6
        Centrioles 7
        Microtubules 7
        Ribosomes 7
        The Endoplasmic Reticulum 7
        Microfilaments 7
        Mitochondria 8
        Lysosomes 8
        Vacuoles 8
        Intracytoplasmic Inclusions 9
        Fundamental Substance 9
    The Cell Membrane 10
        Cilia 10
        Microvilli 12

2. THE NASAL MUCOSA 13
    Microscopic Anatomy
        of the Airway Mucosa 14
    The Epithelial Mucosa 15
    Mucosal Secretion 17
    Mucociliary Transport 18
        Alterations in Mucociliary Transport . . 18
    The Ciliated Cell 19
    The Caliciform Mucous (Goblet) Cell . . . 21
    The Striate Cell 23
    The Basal Cell 24
    The Basal Membrane
    and the Tunica Propria 25

3. INFLAMMATORY CELLS 27
    Morphology and Classification
        of Inflammatory Cells 28
    Neutrophilic Granulocytes 29
    Eosinophilic Granulocytes 32
    Mast Cells 35
    Lymphocytes 39
        Morphologic Classes of Lymphocytes . . 39

        Small Lymphocytes 39
        Large Lymphocytes 39
        Activated Lymphocytes 40
    Functional Classes of Lymphocytes . . . 40
        T Lymphocytes 40
        B Lymphocytes 40
    Plasma Cells 42
    Macrophages 43

4. INFLAMMATORY AGENTS 45
    Pathogenic Microorganisms:
        Bacteria, Fungi and Viruses 46
    Bacteria 47
        Staphylococcus 47
        Streptococcus 47
        Streptococcus Pneumoniae 48
        Diphtheroids 48
        Haemophilus 49
        Moraxella 49
        Neisseria 50
        Pseudomonas 50
    Fungi 51
        Aspergillus 53
        Penicillium 54
        Zygomycetes 54
        Infectious Spot,
            the Morphologic-Chromatic
            Expression of Biofilm 54
    Viruses 57

5. THE LIGHT MICROSCOPE 59
    The Structure of the Light Microscope . . 61
        The Microscope Stand 62
        The Eyepiece 62
        The Objective Lens 63
        Resolving Power 66
        Coverslip 66
        Stage 67
        Substage Condenser 67
        Illuminator 68
        Field Diaphragm 68
    Image Acquisition and Archiving 69

6. CYTOLOGIC PROCEDURES 71
    Equipment and Supplies 73

How to Take a Cytologic Sample......   73
Sampling techniques   74
   Nose Blowing   74
   Nasal Lavage......................   74
   Nasal Swabbing   75
   Nasal Brushing....................   75
   Nasal Scraping   75
   Biopsy   76
Sampling Sites......................   77
Swab Processing   78
Fixation...........................   79
Staining...........................   80
   May-Grünwald-Giemsa (MGG)
   Staining.........................   80
      Effects of MGG Staining.........   81
   Toluidine Blue   82
   Hematoxylin and Eosin Stain (H&E) ..   82
Slide Mounting   84
Slide Destaining   86
Pitfalls and Troubleshooting...........   87
Microscopic Observation   89
   Quantitative Analysis   91
   Semiquantitative Analysis
   and Grading   91

7. **NASAL CYTOPATHOLOGY**...........   95
   Abnormal Cell Processes   96
Degenerative Processes   97
Inflammatory Processes   99
Repair Processes   101
Cytologic Findings in Nasal Diseases....   102
Classification of Rhinitis..............   103
Infectious Rhinitis   104
   Bacterial Rhinitis   104
   Viral Infectious Rhinitis   106
   Fungal Rhinitis...................   109

Inflammatory Rhinitis.................   111
Vasomotor Rhinitis   115
   Allergic Rhinitis...................   115
   Treatment Strategies
   in Allergic Rhinitis   119
   Non Allergic ("Cellular")
   Vasomotor Rhinitis   121
   Non Allergic Rhinitis with Neutrophils
   (NARNE)......................   122
   Non Allergic Rhinitis with Eosinophilia
   Syndrome (NARES)................   123
   Non Allergic Rhinitis with Mast Cells
   (NARMA)   124
   Non Allergic Rhinitis with Eosinophils
   and Mast Cells (NARESMA)   124
   "Overlapping"Rhinopathies   124
   Nasal Cytology in the Diagnostic
   Strategy of Vasomotor Rhinitis   125
Hyperplastic/Granulomatous Rhinitis ..   129
   Nasal-Sinus Polyposis   129
   Clinical-Cytologic Grading
   and Prognostic Index of Relapse......   130
Other Rhinitis   131
   Pregnancy Rhinitis   131
   Rhinitis Medicamentosa.............   131
   Atrophic Rhinitis   131
Conclusion   132

8. **PHOTOMICROGRAPHIC IMAGES
OF NORMAL AND ABNORMAL
NASAL CYTOLOGY**..................   133

REFERENCES.........................   188

INDEX   192

The Cell

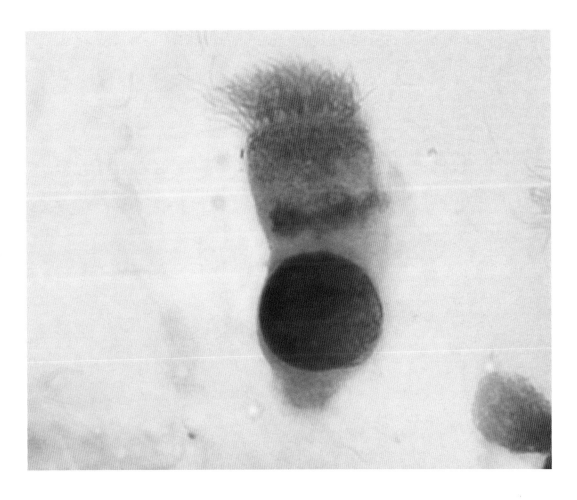

*Now I shall explain how one should treat cellular material
collected for correct microscopic examination,
and I shall describe the methods I myself have tested,
convinced that intelligent individuals
will find others on occasion.*

Henry Baker, 1754

Cell Morphology

The cell is the basic building block of life. It is a self-regulating and self-reproducing biological system that cannot be subdivided.

The cell is composed of two basic components (the *nucleus* and the *cytoplasm*) enclosed within a cell membrane.

A cell's form and volume reflect its function. Free cells such as blood cells are usually spherical, while aggregated cells like epithelial cells have a prismatic-polygonal shape.

Under a light microscope, only a few intracellular structures can be identified even at high magnification (×1000): the nucleus, one or more nucleoli, the cytoplasm, sometimes granules in a variety of shades, and cilia when present.

With the advent of electron microscopy many intracellular organelles were discovered, including mitochondria, the Golgi apparatus, centrioles, microtubules, ribosomes, lysosomes, vacuoles and inclusions, and the nuclear envelope or membrane (**Fig. 1.1**), as well as the fundamental substance in which these structures are suspended. These elements provide the cell with everything it needs to carry out its metabolic functions: maturation and replication, secretion and movement, each of which is finely regulated.

Through research, the specific function of each organelle has been determined, but many other aspects remain to be discovered.

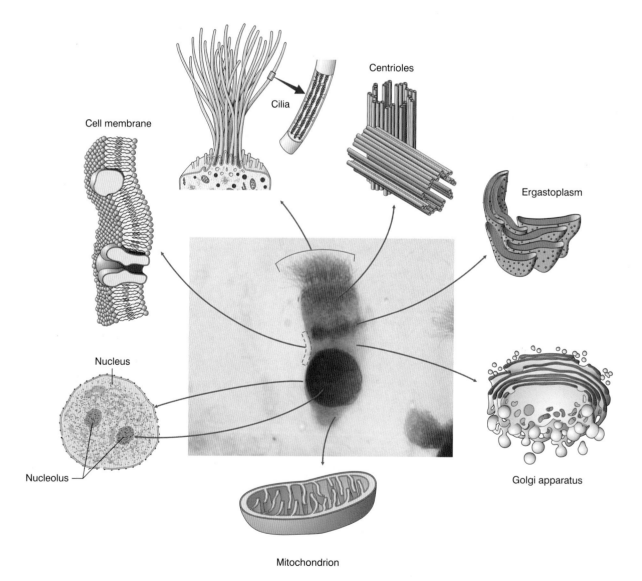

Figure 1.1 Ciliated cell. Intracellular ultrastructural elements.

THE NUCLEUS

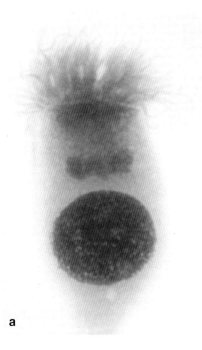 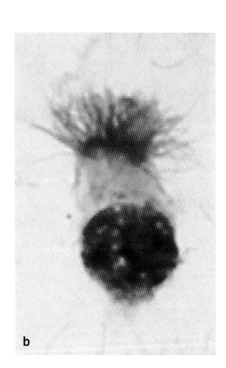

Figure 1.2 Columnar cell of the nasal mucosa. Compact (**a**) and granular (**b**) appearance of the nucleus (MGG staining; ×1000 with a camera magnification factor – CMF – 2×).

The nucleus contains the cell's set of work instructions, controls the fine details of cell synthesis, regulates cell metabolism and supervises the transmission of inheritable traits. In fact, the nucleus contains most of the deoxyribonucleic acid (DNA) responsible for a cell's specific identity.

The ratio between nuclear volume and cytoplasm is fairly constant. During its intermitotic rest phase, the nucleus is composed of four elements: *chromatin, nucleoplasm* or *nuclear fluid, nuclear membrane* and *nucleoli*.

Chromatin

Chromatin varies in appearance, depending on the cell line and growth phase (**Figs. 1.2, 1.3**). The

---

CMF

Camera magnification factor (☞ Chapter 5 – *Image Acquisition and Archiving*).

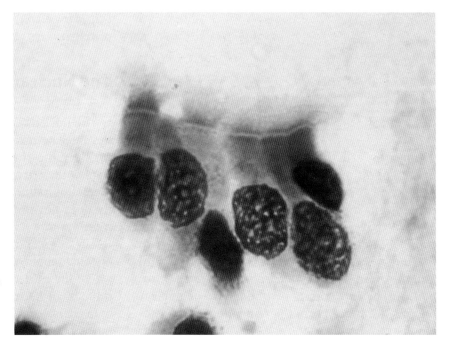

Figure 1.3 Group of ciliated cells of the nasal mucosa in various growth phases (MGG staining; ×1000 with CMF 1×).

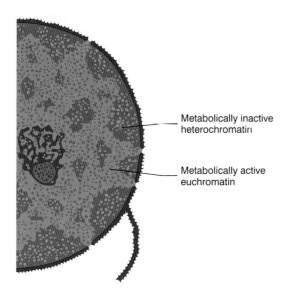

Metabolically inactive heterochromatin

Metabolically active euchromatin

Figure 1.4 Differentiation of nuclear chromatin (reproduction of May-Grümwald-Giemsa – MGG – staining).

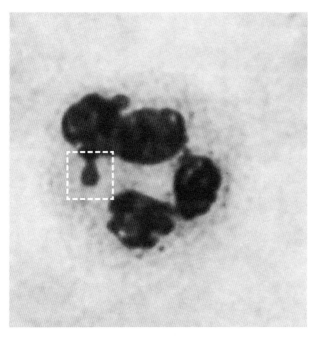

Figure 1.5 Neutrophil with sexual chromatin (inset; MGG staining; ×1000 with CMF 4×).

younger the cell, the more voluminous its nucleus; in this condition, the nucleus-cytoplasm ratio tips in favor of the nucleus, with the chromatin condensed into small granules. By contrast, a mature cell will have dense chromatin clumps forming *chromocenters*. These chromatin clumps adhere to the inner surface of the nuclear membrane and around the nucleolus (*nucleolus-associated chromatin*). They are commonly thought to be nuclear regions not involved in the regulation of cell metabolism.

In the interkinetic phase of the nucleus, only the genetically and hence metabolically inert part of the chromatin (*heterochromatin*) can be readily revealed by histology. The active part (*euchromatin*) is dispersed in the nucleoplasm in this phase (**Fig. 1.4**). This is why in some cases the nuclei of dyskaryotic or malignant cells may appear transparent rather than hyperchromatic, contrary to the tenets of conventional physiopathology.

Sexual chromatin is present in females and appears as a small dense triangular or lentil-shaped mass. In neutrophil granulocytes, sexual chromatin appears as a nuclear appendage (**Fig. 1.5**) and is found in 2-3% of granulocytes. At least 500 cells are needed to be able to determine the genetic sex of an organism. As in Barr bodies, sexual chromatin is the product of the fusion of two X chromosomes. These exteriorize when the nucleus segments.

The Nucleoplasm

The nucleoplasm or *nuclear matrix* can be compared with the *hyaloplasm* (*cytoplasmic matrix*). It appears empty under light microscopy, although high magnification will reveal a thin granulofilamentous web. It may be considered a colloid in which the dispersion or external phase is the fluid and the dispersed or internal phase is made up of protein macromolecules often devoid of enzymatic, metabolic or ionic activity.

The nucleoplasm diminishes with cell senescence, leading to a reduction in nuclear volume. In pathological conditions, the nuclear fluid may increase (*nuclear edema*) or condense and disappear completely (*nuclear pyknosis*) (**Fig. 1.6**).

The Nuclear Membrane

The nucleus is surrounded by an envelope called the nuclear membrane. This structure undergoes considerable change depending on the functional state of the cell and is continuous with the lumen of the endoplasmic reticulum; however, this continuity does not prevent the nucleus from moving or rotating.

The nuclear membrane is perforated by round openings about 50 μm in diameter, the *nuclear pores*, where the nucleoplasm and the cytoplasm are continuous. In normal conditions, the pores are closed by a diaphragm, in front of which there is always nucleoplasm but never chromocenters. In certain

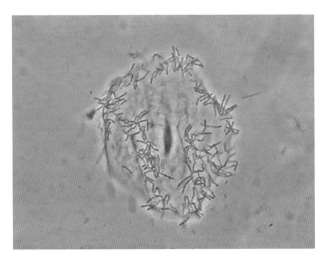

Figure 1.6 Squamous epithelial cell of the nasal vestibule with pyknotic nucleus (phase-contrast microscopy). Numerous bacteria are adherent to the cell surface (bacterial adhesion) (×1000 with CMF 1.4×).

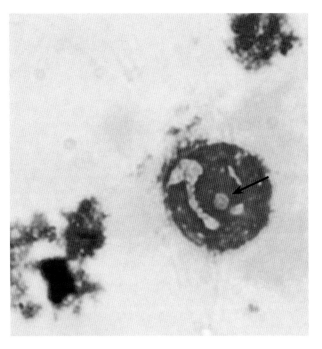

Figure 1.7 Bare nucleus with prominent nucleolus (arrow) (MGG staining; ×1000).

cells, the nuclear pores account for 10% of the membrane surface area; in others the pores may be far fewer. As a rule, the number of pores decreases with cell age.

The Nucleolus

The nucleolus is an intranuclear area where ribonucleic acid (RNA) is synthesized, therefore it is more pronounced in active or reactive cells.

One or more nucleoli may be present in a nucleus and their position and volume vary greatly.

The characteristic intense blue staining (*basophilia*) (**Fig. 1.7**) depends on the amount of RNA they contain. Sometimes they may be colorless but can still be seen owing to the presence of a thick chromatin strip along their edges; sometimes they may be completely hidden by nucleolus-associated chromocenters. It is to be noted that cell malignancy is not indicated by the presence of one nucleolus or

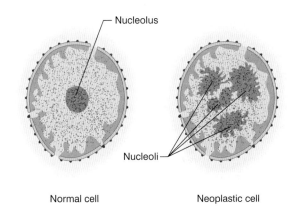

Normal cell   Neoplastic cell

Figure 1.8 Enlarged, multiple nucleoli with irregular borders are signs indicating malignancy.

several small nucleoli, but rather by the presence of abnormally large, irregular or numerous nucleoli (**Fig. 1.8**).

THE CYTOPLASM

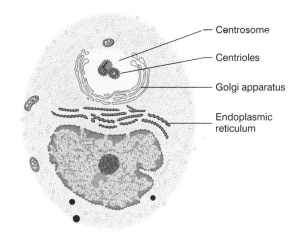

Figure 1.9 Area of the centrosome containing the organelles.

The cytoplasm constitutes the cell's inner environment. It is composed of water, organic molecules and ions and provides the basic substances needed for the chemical reactions in cell metabolism.

Under light microscopy the *cytoplasmic matrix* appears homogenous and contains nearly unidentifiable inclusion bodies. Electron microscopy reveals organelles and other fine structures.

Smears will display an area of clear cytoplasm without granules: the *centrosome* or cytocentrum. This is composed of the *Golgi apparatus*, which de-

limits the space where the *centrioles* are located (**Fig. 1.9**). Since the mass of the centrosome is more resistant than that of the nucleus, the latter yields to the stiffness of the centrosome, becoming kidney-shaped or sometimes even bilobed. The depression in the nucleus is thus due to the presence of the centrosome (**Fig. 1.10**).

This region is characterized by a rhythmic beating motion that is thought to circulate material and organelles within the cytoplasm. This motion ceases at low temperatures or when the cell enters apoptosis.

The Golgi Apparatus

The Golgi apparatus is composed of dictyosomes that are more or less extensively connected with each other, so as to form a hollow sphere, within which are contained the *centrioles* (**Fig. 1.11**).

Each dictyosome is composed of a series (2-8) of flattened sacs.

These sacs are nearly empty when the cell is at metabolic rest. In the active phase, the dictyosomes separate and the numerous vesicles containing metabolic products (e.g. gamma globulin, specific granules, lysosomes) detach from their borders. The dictyosomes also contain a variety of enzymes that catalyze mucopolysaccharide and saccharide metabolism.

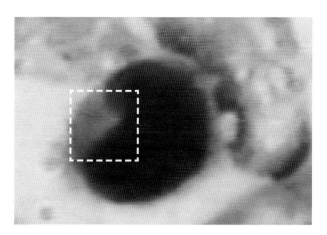

Figure 1.10 Lymphocyte. Transparent area corresponding to the centrosome or cytocentrum (inset) represents the more rigid part of the cytoskeleton. The nucleus loses its rigidity in the cytocentrum, forming a nuclear notch (MGG staining; ×1000 with CMF 4×).

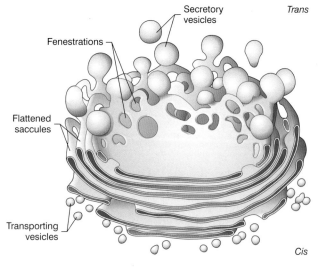

Figure 1.11 Ultrastructure of the Golgi apparatus.

Centrioles

Two centrioles are present in the cell at mitotic rest (**Fig. 1.12**). They resemble small tubular structures (150 μm in diameter; 300-500 μm in length) arranged so that the longitudinal axis of one is perpendicular to that of the other. The walls are composed of nine groups of three tubules each in a helical arrangement.

Centrioles intervene in mitosis and cell movement. At the end of cell division, they self-replicate.

Microtubules

Microtubules are tubular structures (about 200 μm across, of variable length and having walls about 4 μm thick) formed by 13 filaments composed of spheres of equal diameter. They form a type of cytoskeleton that lends shape to the cell.

During mitosis, the microtubules form spindle fibers.

During telophase, they gather in the area where the two cells separate and the two daughter cells then remain connected by a mitotic bridge for a certain period.

Ribosomes

Ribosomes are granules (about 140 Å in diameter) present in all cells except red blood cells and consisting primarily of RNA and proteins.

They are composed of two subunits differing in molecular weight (40 and 60 S). They can be found in the nucleus, the nucleoli and particularly in the cytoplasm where their amount determines the degree of basophilia of the cell. They receive messenger RNA (mRNA) and transfer RNA (tRNA) and play an important role in protein synthesis.

In the cytoplasm, ribosomes can be isolated (*monoribosomes*), grouped (3-10 elements) or clustered (*polyribosomes*) in larger groups connected by a thin filament of mRNA.

Ribosomes can be found adhering to the outer surface of the *endoplasmic reticulum*.

The Endoplasmic Reticulum

The endoplasmic reticulum (ER) is a loose network of cytoplasmic tubules and flattened sacs with (rough ER) or without (smooth ER) ribosomes on the surface of their membranes (**Fig. 1.13**).

Inside the endoplasmic reticulum the substances processed by the ribosomes, generally proteins, ac-

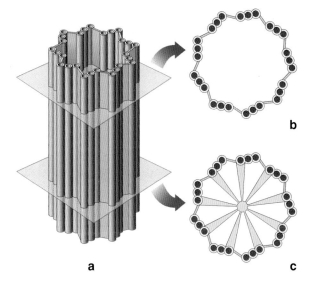

Figure 1.12 Centrioles. Tridimensional model (**a**); section through the proximal part (nine triplets) (**b**); section through the distal part (cart wheel) (**c**).

cumulate and move to other areas of the cell, mainly to the Golgi apparatus.

Under light microscopy, smooth ER is invisible, while rough ER, when arranged in sufficiently large piles, appears as a blue multilayered structure that cytologists once termed *ergastoplasm* or granular endoplasmic reticulum.

Microfilaments

Microfilaments generally appear as fibrils or fibril groups (about 5 μ in diameter) often arranged

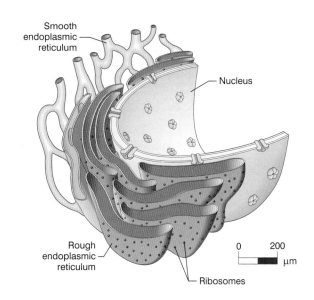

Smooth endoplasmic reticulum

Nucleus

Rough endoplasmic reticulum

Ribosomes

0   200
μm

Figure 1.13 Rough endoplasmic reticulum.

around the nucleus or close to the nuclear membrane and consisting primarily of actinomyosin.

They play an important role in cellular and intercellular movement. They are invisible under light microscopy.

Mitochondria

Mitochondria are round or oval or rod-shaped structures (5-10 µm to 40 µm long and 0.5-1 µm wide).

Each cell has a fairly constant number of mitochondria, although this number can differ widely from one cell line to another. During the stages of the cell cycle, the number increases as the cell matures.

This organelle consists of two sets of equally thick membranes, an outer coat and an inner membrane arranged in folds that form the *cristae* where the enzymes are located that supply the cell with its energy (ATP) (**Fig. 1.14**). Inside the mitochondrion is a substance composed of proteins, phospholipids, ribosomes and some DNA in the *mitochondrial chromosome.*

Mitochondria are invisible under a light microscope. In intensely stained cytoplasm, they can be located by their negative image.

Lysosomes

Lysosomes are granulations containing proteolytic enzymes. These are activated on rupture of the lysosomal membrane, which generally occurs in a vacuole of phagocytosis.

Lysosomal enzymes come in a wide variety, including ribonuclease, deoxyribonuclease, and over twenty types of hydrolytic enzymes. Under light and electron microscopy, lysosomes can usually be identified by their reaction with esterase and acid phosphatase.

Secondary lysosomes are vacuoles resulting from the fusion of lysosomes and phagosomes, or autophagolysosomes. Under light microscopy, they often appear as granules, although many cannot be visualized.

Specific leukocytic granulations are particular lysosomes whose content is specific to a cell line and may be distinguished as *neutrophilic*, *eosinophilic* or *basophilic* granulations (**Fig. 1.15**).

Vacuoles

Vacuoles can be divided into:
* *contractile* vacuoles resembling protozoan contractile vacuoles;
* *lipid* vacuoles, which are rare in the normal physiologic states but may be seen frequently in many pathologic conditions and during cell aging *in vivo*;
* *multivesicular* bodies that probably derive from pinocytosis. Their function is still unknown.

When large enough to be visible under light mi-

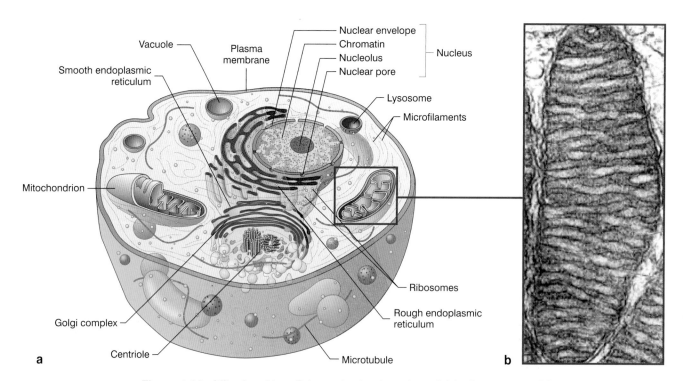

Figure 1.14 Mitochondrion. Schematic drawing of a cell (**a**); ultrastructure (**b**).

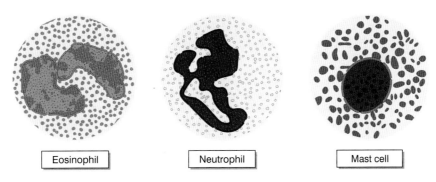

Figure 1.15 Lysosomal granules can be colored with special stains (reproduction of May-Grünwald-Giemsa – MGG – staining).

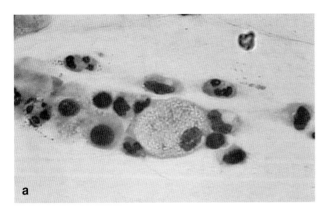
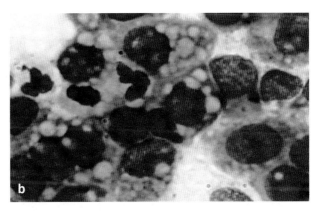

Figure 1.16 a, b Cells with numerous intracytoplasmic vacuoles (MGG staining; **a**, ×1000; **b**, ×1000 with CMF 2.2×)

croscopy, these structures appear as empty spaces on slide smears (**Fig. 1.16 a-b**).

Intracytoplasmic Inclusions

Inclusions are secretory deposits temporarily stored by the cell. They can contain a wide variety of substances, including proteins, hemosiderin, and mucopolysaccharides. In pathologic conditions, they can populate the entire cytoplasm (**Fig. 1.17**).

Under light microscopy, they can be demonstrated only by specific fixation and staining; May-Grünwald-Giemsa (MGG) staining dissolves most of them.

Fundamental Substance

Fundamental substance is the space between cellular organelles where no structures can be identified with current methods of observation. Fundamental substance is composed of water and soluble molecules that disappear with the use of conven-

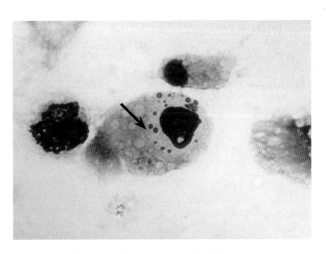

Figure 1.17 Ciliated columnar cell of the nasal mucosa with signs of ciliocytophthoria: numerous intracytoplasmic vacuoles and nuclear chromatin both in dispersed (arrow) and aggregated form are visible (MGG staining; ×1000 with CMF 1.2×).

tional fixation and inclusion techniques. It plays a major role in cell physiology and pathology since it constitutes the microenvironment that contains the organelles and coordinates their functioning.

THE CELL MEMBRANE

By revealing the fine structure of the cell, electron microscopy has improved our knowledge of the cell membrane (about 8 μm thick).

Like all biological membranes, it is composed of two phospholipid layers between which proteins are located. Its function cannot be fully appreciated without considering the interactions between its inward facing layer which contains enzymes and contractile proteins, and its outer layer containing receptors and molecules that determine the specific nature of the cell.

The particular structure of the cell membrane enables it to carry out three essential functions:

- it regulates exchanges with the external environment (e.g. selective permeability, endocytosis, exocytosis, locomotion);
- it receives hormonal and other signals that regulate its function;
- it bears specific attributes (blood group, tissue traits, various receptors) that render the cell recognizable to other cells.

Light microscopy can demonstrate major changes in the cell membrane but not show other characteristics common to nearly all cells such as microvilli and microinvaginations.

Cilia

The cilia (5-10 μm long and 0.2 μm across) are motile extensions of the cell surface closely related to the centrioles. They play a predominantly kinetic (*vibratory cilia*) but sometimes a sensory role. They can vary in number. In the tracheal epithelium a single cell may have up to 200-250 cilia compared to about 100 per cell in the nasal epithelium. Generally, each cilium is formed by a flexible extension from the cell membrane containing scarce hyaloplasm (**Figs. 1.18-1.20**).

Under ultramicroscopy, the cilia are composed of an array of nine double microtubules arranged in a peripheral ring surrounding a central pair (9+2). The subunits are composed of a bundle of 11-12

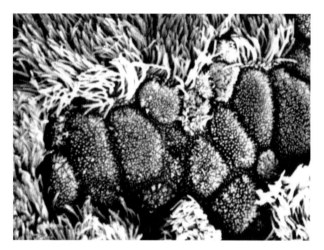

Figure 1.18 Ciliated cells (scanning electron microscopy).

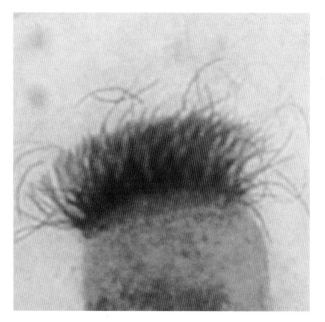

Figure 1.19 Ciliary apparatus (MGG staining; ×1000 with CMF 4×).

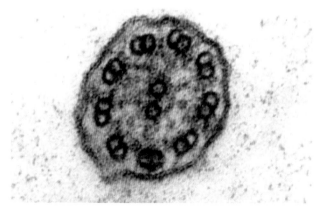

Figure 1.20 Ciliary ultrastructure (electron microscopy).

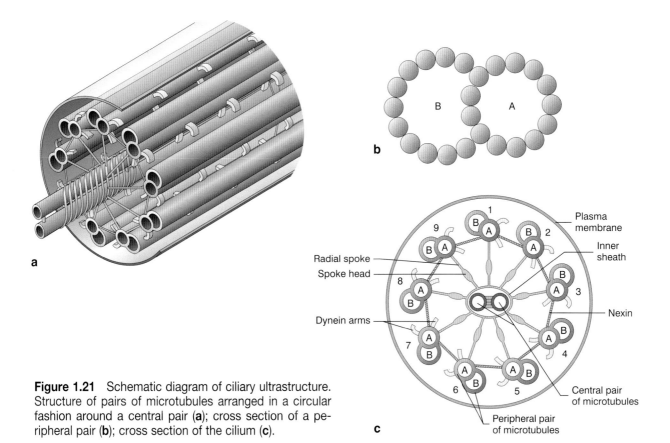

Figure 1.21 Schematic diagram of ciliary ultrastructure. Structure of pairs of microtubules arranged in a circular fashion around a central pair (**a**); cross section of a peripheral pair (**b**); cross section of the cilium (**c**).

protofilaments consisting of globular stacks (**Fig. 1.21 a-b**).

In animal and plant cells, this microtubular architecture is constant in all cilia, except in rare instances. Each pair of peripheral microtubules is composed of a subfiber A, which has two side arms orientated clockwise, and a subfiber B. The subfibers are fused together, while the microtubules of the central pair are separate and held together by a helical sheath (**Fig. 1.21 c**).

At the base of each cilia, the nine pairs of peripheral tubules are connected by a centriolar structure, the *basal corpuscle*, while the central pair disappears. At the other end of the basal corpuscle, fibrilar structures (*root of cilia*) with a periodic band (about 50-70 µm) penetrate into the cell. Besides tubulin, a microtubule protein, the cilia contain a special protein (*dinein*) rich in ATP-ase.

Ciliary motion begins at the root of the cilia. The cilia move rapidly in coordinated movements produced by the sliding of the microtubules against one another and characterized by a rapid impulse that produces propulsive movement and a slow impulse that generates the return movement (**Fig. 1.22**).

At their tip the cilia have small club-shaped projections about 25-60 nm thick that wave synchronic-ally at a frequency of about 600-1000 beats per minute, moving in the same direction but with a slightly delayed phase. This is called *metachronous movement*.

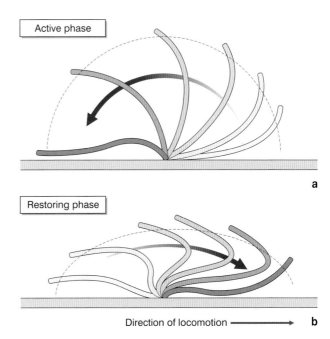

Figure 1.22 Ciliary beat. Rapid or active phase (**a**); slow or restoring phase (**b**).

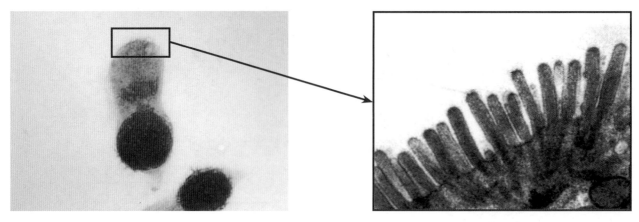

Figure 1.23 Striate cell with microvilli at its apex (insert: electron microscopic view; MGG staining; ×1000 with CMF 1.2×).

Microvilli

Microvilli are appendages on the cell membrane differing in length and usually cylindrical in shape (**Fig. 1.23**). Their number differs in many types of cells; their purpose is to augment the free cell surface area, thus augmenting the exchange between the external environment and the internal world of the cell.

The microvilli are not precursors to the cilia; they preserve the moisture needed for ciliary function and inhibit surface dehydration.

The Nasal Mucosa

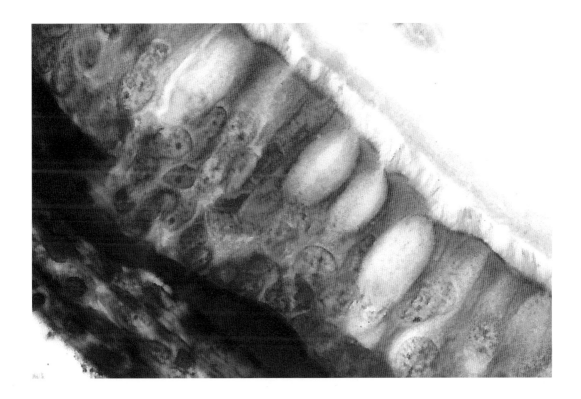

The teacher's role is not just to teach facts but to stimulate new ways of thinking.

Albert Policard, 1962

Microscopic Anatomy of the Airway Mucosa

The nasal cavity extends from the nares anteriorly to its termination posteriorly at the choana, where its opens into the nasopharynx.

Each side of the nasal cavity has two parts: the *vestibule*, in front, and the true *nasal cavity*. The latter contains the *olfactory cleft* (*pars olfactoria*) and the *paranasal sinuses* (ethmoid cells, frontal, maxillary and sphenoid sinuses) that drain into it (**Fig. 2.1**).

The respiratory portion of the nasal fossae and wide sections of the olfactory cleft are covered by a smooth pink mucosal lining about 2 μm thick. In some portions, this mucosa adheres to the perichondrium, in others to the periostium. The mucosal lining becomes thicker (up to 3-5 μm) at the level of the inferior turbinate where it is rich in cavernous tissue, especially on the convex surface. The mucosa is thinner over the middle turbinate except at the

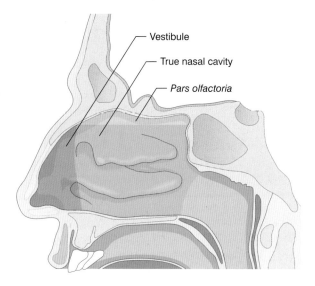

Figure 2.1 Areas of the nasal cavity.

free edge of the head and tail where it thickens again due to the presence of cavernous vascular tissue (**Fig. 2.2**).

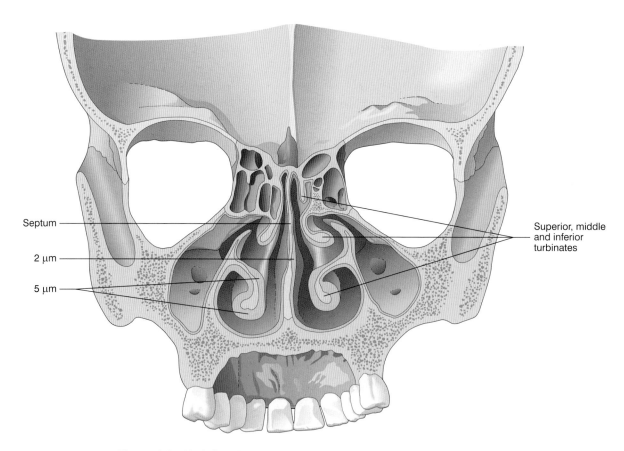

Figure 2.2 Variations in mucosal thickness inside the nasal cavity.

THE EPITHELIAL MUCOSA

Microscopically, the nasal mucosa consists of an epithelium resting on a thin basal membrane that separates it from the tunica propria. The pseudostratified columnar epithelium is composed of ciliated and non ciliated columnar cells (also called brush border or striate cells), mucous caliciform cells (also called *goblet cells*) and basal cells (**Fig. 2.3 a-b**). All these cells are closely interconnected through desmoidal and hemidesmoidal junction systems. Lymphocytes and polymorphonucleates can sometimes be observed in the intercellular spaces.

Although the epithelial mucosa is generally considered to be a mere physical barrier between the organism and irritating agents (chemical, physical, bacterial and viral agents), it is, in fact, metabolically active. For instance, in immune inflammatory reactions it plays an important role in regulating host response, producing a wide variety of inhibitors such as proteases (elafin, secretory leukocyte protease inhibitor [SLPI]) and the secretory component of IgA.

Within the nasal cavity, the epithelial mucosa displays several histologic differences depending on the site examined (**Fig. 2.4**).

The nasal vestibule is covered with skin which, at the rim of the nostril, is continuous with the skin of the external nose, while toward the nasal cavity it transitions into the respiratory mucosa. The skin of the vestibule is thin and composed of *keratinized stratified squamous epithelium* (**Fig. 2.5**). The epi-

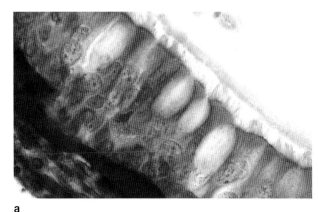

a

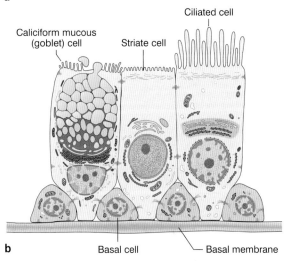

b

Figure 2.3 Respiratory mucosa as it appears in a histological preparation (**a**). Cell types of the nasal mucosa (**b**).

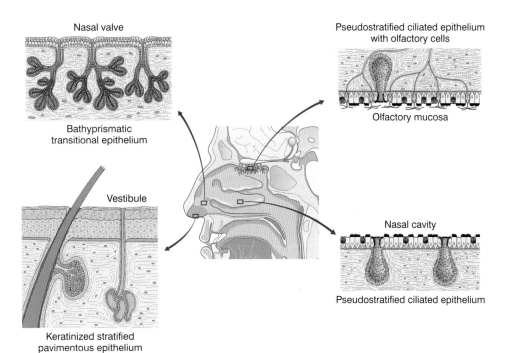

Figure 2.4 Histologic features of the nasal mucosa in different areas of the nasal cavity.

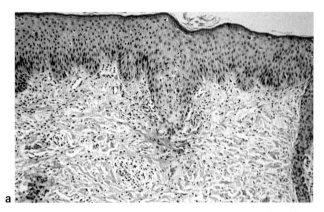

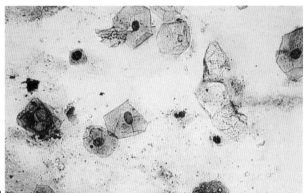

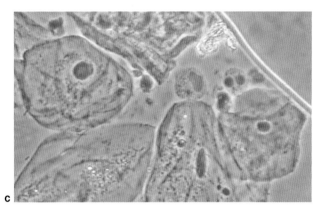

Figure 2.5 Histologic (**a**) and cytologic aspects of a sample taken from the epithelium of the nasal vestibule (**b**, **c**). Squamous epithelial cells of the nasal vestibule seen at light microscopy (**b**) and phase-contrast microscopy (**c**).

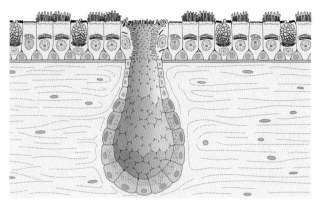

Figure 2.6 Tubuloacinar glands of the respiratory mucosa.

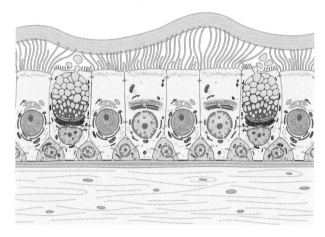

Figure 2.7 Pseudostratified ciliated columnar epithelium of the nasal mucosa.

thelium comprises different parts, including robust rigid hairs, termed *vibrissae*, voluminous sebaceous glands and small eccrine and apocrine sweat glands (*vestibular glands*).

The epithelium of the vestibule then gives way to the *transitional epithelium*. At this border area with the respiratory mucosa, the epithelium replaces its outer layer with a *stratified bathyprismatic epithelium*; the vibrissae, sebaceous and sweat glands disappear while in the tunica propria the *compound tubuloacinar glands*, characteristic of the respiratory mucosa, appear (**Fig. 2.6**).

The remaining portion of the nasal mucosa, starting at the area anterior to the head of the inferior turbinate and excluding the upper part covered by the olfactory epithelium, is composed of the *pseudostratified ciliated columnar epithelium*.

An appreciation of these histologic differences is extremely useful in clinical practice. For example the presence, in a rhinocytogram, of unexpected cell types (e.g. squamous cells of the epithelium of the vestibule) immediately shows that the sample was incorrectly taken.

It should be emphasized here that while the term *pseudostratified* refers to the fact that the nuclei of these cells are located at different heights, leaving the observer with the impression of an epithelium arranged in different layers, high-power light microscopy and electron microscopy have shown that all cell types are in direct contact with the basal lamina, although not all reach the surface of the epithelium (**Fig. 2.7**).

MUCOSAL SECRETION

An additional attribute of the respiratory epithelium is the mucous that covers the entire epithelial surface. Microscopically, the mucous is arranged in two overlapping layers (*sol-gel*). The layer in direct contact with the epithelial surface is fluid (*sol phase*), and about 3 μm thick. The cilia of the epithelial cells are nearly completely submerged in this. This acqueous stratum is generated by the polarized transport of solutes by the epithelial cells.

Above the hydrosaline layer generated by the epithelium lies a dense layer (*gel*), about 5 μm thick, composed primarily of glycoproteins called *mucins*. These glycoproteins present a central protein structure in which polysaccharide side chains consisting of syalic acid (*syalomucin*) or fucose (*fucomucin*) or sulfur groups (*sulfomucin*) are anchored.

These glycoproteins are produced by the goblet cells and the submucosal glands. The latter synthesize about 40 times the amount synthesized by the superficial goblet cells.

MUCOCILIARY TRANSPORT

The two mucous (sol-gel) layers constitute an important non specific defense system of the upper airways that decontaminates inhaled air. Inspired particles, whether inert or consisting of microorganisms, collide with the gel layer and remain trapped. Airflow turbulence helps in this process.

The sol phase of the secretion permits appropriate movement of the cilia which, on straightening, grasp the gel layer with their tips, propelling it toward the nasopharynx where it is eliminated. Conversely, there does not seem to be any propulsion of the sol layer.

The cilia propel the gel layer in rhythmic movements at a mean frequency of about 800 beats per minute which differs slightly in various areas of the airway tract. This sliding of the gel over the sol is enhanced by a thin layer of predominantly monomolecular phospholipids at the gel-sol interface.

Alterations in Mucociliary Transport

Given the complexity of the mucociliary transport system, the causes of impaired mucous *clearance* can be deduced by examining its components.

Table 2.1 Bacteria commonly causing ciliary dyskinesia

- *Pseudomonas aeruginosa*
- *Haemophilus influenzae*
- *Staphylococcus aureus*
- *Streptococcus pneumoniae*
- *Mycoplasma pneumoniae*
- *Neisseria meningitidis*
- *Neisseria gonorrhoeae*

Mucociliary clearance may be altered by changes in ciliary motility, in the periciliary fluid (sol phase), in the gel layer or in the monomolecular phospholipid layer at the gel-sol interface.

Other conditions that may impair ciliary function include primary (e.g. immotile cilia syndrome associated, or not, with *situs viscerum inversus*) or secondary causes. Some secondary causes include viral or bacterial infections (**Table 2.1**) and inhalation of environmental toxins and/or tobacco smoke which can lead to lysis of ciliated cells or secondary ciliary dyskinesia.

In such circumstances, the mucosal secretion will tend to accumulate and thicken, forming mucosal plugs or crusts.

More complex and less known alterations involve the components of the secretion itself. Changes in the secretion and reabsorption of periciliary fluid can alter the sol layer thickness. The consequences are:

- increased sol phase thickness which prevents the cilia from grasping the gel layer, causing the cilia to vibrate uselessly;
- decreased sol phase thickness which promotes persistent anchoring of the cilia in the gel layer, engulfing the cilia in the gel.

In both situations, effective propulsion of the gel layer is inhibited.

This is also why inhaling air that is too dry can decrease the sol thickness of the secretion, resulting in altered mucosal clearance.

Studies that investigate the mechanisms underlying the production and reabsorption of periciliary fluid, and those directed at identifying the regulatory centers of mucin and surfactant production in normal and pathologic conditions, will best enable us to understand the pathophysiology of alterations in the mucociliary *clearance* system and permit more efficacious approaches to treatment.

THE CILIATED CELL

The ciliated cell is the most differentiated and the most numerous cell type, accounting for about 80% of the cells making up the nasal mucosa.

The ratio between ciliated and non ciliated cells is 5:1 and increases proceeding distally toward the lower airways where it peaks at 100-200:1.

Each ciliated cell is flanked by non ciliated cells and has submucosal gland ducts. Ciliated cells are elongated polygons, 15-20 µm tall, with nuclei located at various heights above the basal membrane, giving the epithelial mucosa its typical pseudostratified appearance under microscopy. The top surface is composed of about 100-250 cilia (each 10-15 µm long and 0.2 µm across) (**Fig. 2.8**) and about 300 microvilli.

On a nasal cytogram, the ciliated cell displays a typical morphology (**Fig. 2.9**) owing to its location in the epithelium.

At a magnification of at least ×400, the cell surface can be seen, consisting of the ciliary apparatus, a distinct structure that comprises most of the cytoplasm, and the nucleus. The basal region, which we could call the "foot" of the ciliated cell, is tapered where it comes into contact with the basal membrane (**Fig. 2.10**). Electron microscopic studies have shown that the ciliated cell is not anchored to the basal membrane; instead, it is attached to the tunica propria at junction sites of the desmosomes with the basal cells.

The same holds true for goblet and striated cells, which are separated from the basal membrane by a layer of *laminin*, a cellular adhesion molecule (**Fig. 2.11**).

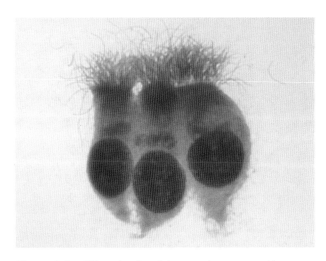

Figure 2.8 Ciliated cells of the nasal mucosa with prominent ciliary apparatus.

A study we conducted showed that inside the cytoplasm of ciliated columnar cells stained with MGG there is a hyperchromatic line above the nucleus. We termed this the *supranuclear hyperchromatic stria* (SHS) (**Fig. 2.12 a-b**).

This line is selectively present in cells not affected by cellular alterations of the nucleus, cytoplasm or ciliary apparatus; hence, it gives a direct indication of cellular integrity.

This was confirmed by the observation of a statistically significant reduction in the proportion of cells demonstrating a stria (SHS+) in vasomotor, inflammatory and infectious nasal diseases. Furthermore, the proportion of cells without striae correlated with the severity of the disease.

It is thought that the stria is the staining ex-

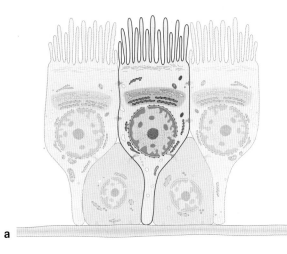

Figure 2.9 Ciliated cell. Schematic drawing representing a ciliated cell within the epithelial mucosa (**a**); isolated ciliated cell (**b**). MGG staining; ×1000 with CMF 2×).

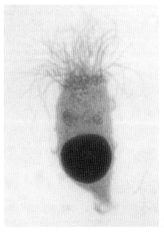

a

b

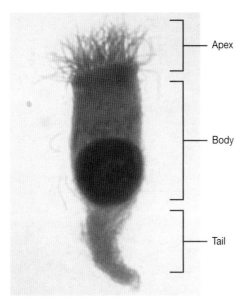

Figure 2.10 Regions of the ciliated cell (MGG staining; ×1000 with CMF 2×).

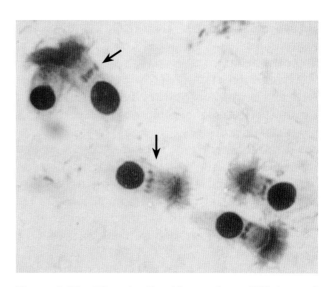

Figure 2.11 Only the laminin layer separates the basal membrane from ciliated, striate and goblet cells.

pression of the rough endoplasmic reticulum or Golgi apparatus. Electron microscopic and cell biochemistry studies are investigating this hypothesis. The stria can easily be seen in metabolically active cells (**Fig. 2.13**) but not in altered cells (**Fig. 2.14**).

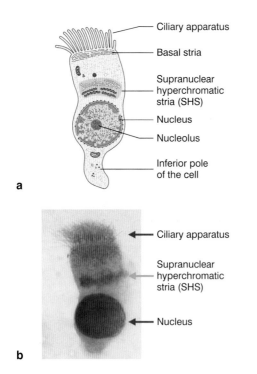

Figure 2.12 Ciliated cell with prominent supranuclear hyperchromatic stria (SHS) (**a**). Cytologic appearance (**b**).

Figure 2.13 Ciliated cells with prominent SHS (arrows) (MGG staining; ×1000).

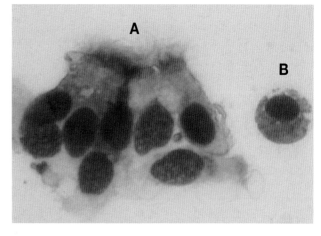

Figure 2.14 Ciliated cells with negative SHS (A); eosinophil (B) (MGG staining; ×1000 with CMF 1.2×).

THE CALICIFORM MUCOUS (GOBLET) CELL

The *goblet cell* or mucous cell (**Fig. 2.15**) is a unicellular gland set between the cells of the pseudostratified respiratory epithelium. This gland secretes a viscous fluid, or *mucin*, a polysaccharide protein that, combined with water, forms mucus.

The surface of the goblet cell is covered with numerous microvilli that differ in size depending on the stage of cell secretion. It has a small opening, the *stoma*, through which mucin granules spill out by exocytosis onto the epithelial surface.

The mucocytic granules contain mostly neutral mucin, syalomucin and sulfomucin, unlike serous cells which produce a less viscous secretion rich in neutral glycoproteins, lysosomes and an IgA epithelial transfer element.

The nucleus is located at the base of the cell, while the vacuoles containing the *mucinogenic* granules, biochemical precursors of mucin, are located above the nucleus, giving the mature cell its characteristic goblet form.

As with ciliated cells, only the tapered end of the basal cytoplasm rests on the basal membrane.

As the amount of mucus increases and the nucleus is pushed downward, a characteristic area of dense chromatin forms that is evident on common cytologic preparations, making goblet cells easily recognizable (**Fig. 2.16**), even though the intracytoplasmic content often appears empty under light microscopy because the mucus granules are degraded by common fixation methods (**Fig. 2.17**).

Goblet cells play a highly important physiological role because their secretion in the respiratory tract is essential for maintaining adequate airway clearance.

In humans, the density of goblet cells increases up to adolescence.

Although they normally account for only 1% of the total number of epithelial cells in the respiratory tract, their number can increase considerably when the airways are chronically exposed to irritants (**Figs. 2.18 a-b**, **2.19**).

There are no goblet cells in the squamous, transitional or olfactory epithelia. They are irregularly distributed in the pseudostratified mucosal epithelium. In areas where the nasal glands are more scarce, goblet cells are the main source for the formation of the mucosal lining of the respiratory surface.

In the septal region, goblet cells are less densely

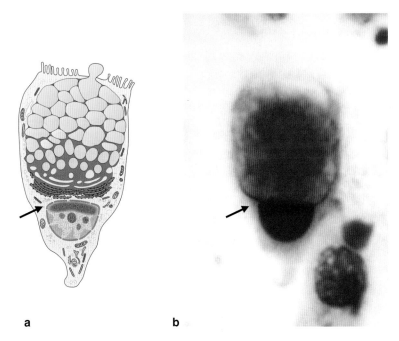

a   b

Figure 2.15 Goblet cell. Schematic drawing (**a**); cytologic apperance (**b**). The arrow shows the chromatic enhancement of the nuclear chromatin (MGG staining; ×1000 with CMF 2×).

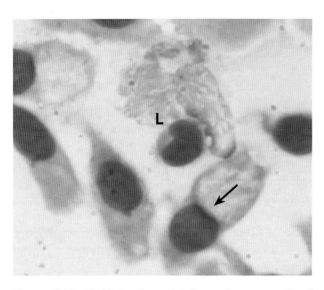

Figure 2.16 Goblet cells containing various amounts of cytoplasm. Condensed chromatin (arrow) resulting from mucin pressing on the nucleus. Lymphocyte (L) seen at the center of the microscopic field (MGG staining; ×1000 with CMF 1.4×).

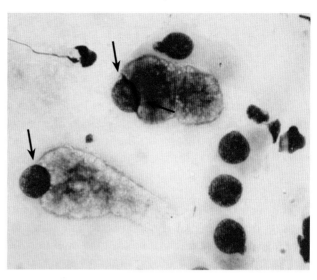

Figure 2.17 Goblet cells with evident chromatic enhancement of nuclear chromatin (arrows) (MGG staining; ×1000 with CMF 1.2×).

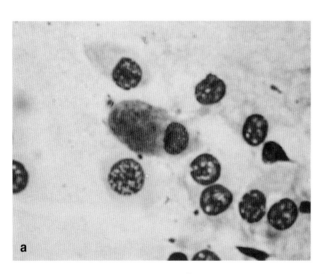
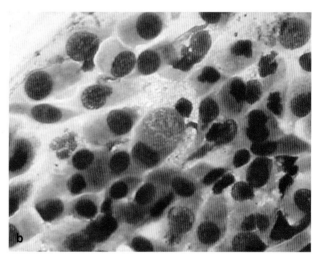

Figure 2.18 a, b Goblet cell in the center of the microscopic field (MGG staining; ×1000).

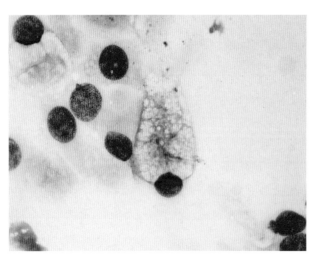

Figure 2.19 Goblet cell (MGG staining; ×1000 with CMF 1.2×).

distributed than in the turbinates. The middle turbinate has the lowest goblet cell density. The goblet cell population gradually decreases in the more inferior and more posterior tissues.

THE STRIATE CELL

Like ciliated and goblet cells, the striate cell is a columnar cell with its nucleus located toward the inferior pole.

Ultrastructural studies show a cell membrane surface with a uniform series of raised microvilli, in the center of which are microfilaments. Additional microfilaments form bundles within in the cytoplasm adjacent to the cisternae of the rough endoplasmic reticulum, and abundant glycogenic granulations (**Fig. 2.20 a-b**).

The function of these cells is unclear. They are thought to be absorbent cells for chemoreceptors or perhaps precursor cells of ciliated cells, but no evidence supporting this hypothesis has been found (**Fig. 2.21**).

As mentioned in the previous chapter, the microvilli augment cell surface area, inhibit dehydration of the mucosal surface, and maintain adequate moisture necessary for ciliary function.

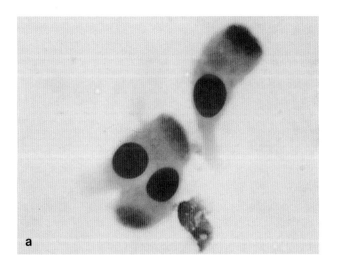
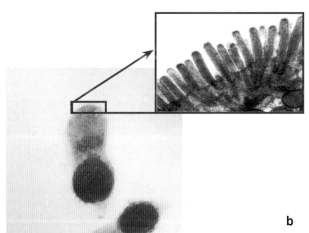

Figure 2.20 Group of striate cells (**a**). Ultramicroscopic view showing microvilli at the cell apex (inset) (**b**) (MGG staining; ×1000 with CMF 1.2×).

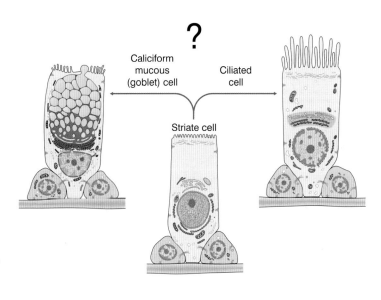

Figure 2.21 Hypothetically, striate cells differentiate into ciliated and/or goblet cells.

THE BASAL CELL

So called because it adheres to the basal membrane, this relatively small cell does not reach the superficial layer of the airways. It has an electrodense cytoplasm with tonofilament bundles, few mitochondria, scarce rough endoplasmic reticulum and a large nucleus that is hyperchromatic with respect to the cytoplasm (**Fig. 2.22 a-b**).

Basal cells were long believed to be the precursors of the goblet and epithelial cells of the airways, but the data supporting this belief remain controversial.

It appears that basal cells promote the adhesion of columnar cells to the basal membrane. This is confirmed by the fact that columnar cells have no hemidesmosomal junctions and are attached to the basal membrane by cell adhesion molecules. Moreover, the number of basal cells correlates positively with the height of columnar cells in the airways; thus the taller the columnar cells, the smaller the contact area with the basal membrane and the greater the number of basal cells that ensure adhesion of the columnar cells (**Fig. 2.23 a-b**).

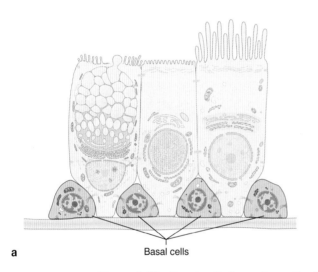

a

Basal cells

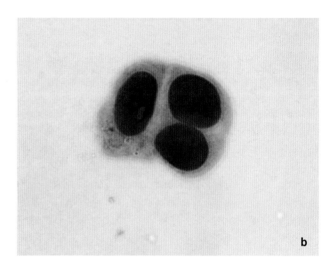

b

Figure 2.22 Basal cells in a schematic diagram (**a**) and in a cytologic preparation (**b**).

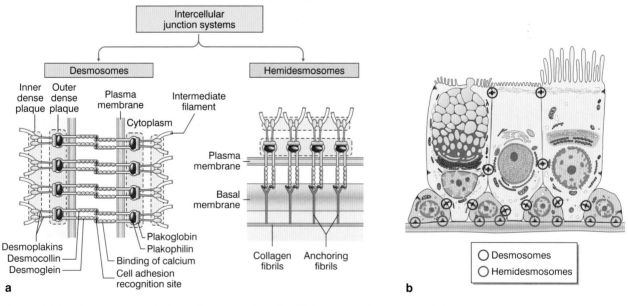

a

b

Figure 2.23 Electron transmission microscopy has shed light on certain aspects of the function of intercellular adhesion junctions (desmosomes and hemidesmosomes). Structural details of the junctional apparatus (**a**); localization of the junctional apparatus (**b**).

THE BASAL MEMBRANE AND THE TUNICA PROPRIA

The respiratory epithelium is separated from the tunica propria by the basal membrane, a thin hyaline membrane (0.2 μm thick) perforated by openings through which leukocytes migrate toward the epithelial surface; it is highly resistant and strongly adherent to the epithelial cells.

The *tunica propria*, or *stroma* or *chorion*, is composed of fibroelastic connective tissue on which the epithelium rests and extends to the periostium and perichondrium.

The basal membrane has three layers:
- the subepithelial or lymphoid layer;
- the intermediate or glandular layer;
- the deep layer or vascular layer zone (**Fig. 2.24**).

The *subepithelial layer* lying beneath the basal membrane is relatively lax and rich in lymphocytes (hence the term *lymphoid*), which are often arranged in nodules (*nasal-associated lymphoid tissue*, NALT), especially in the posterior portion of the nasal cavity.

The *intermediate layer* is rich in glandular bodies. Their secretion has an anti-infectious action owing to the presence of lysozyme and immunoglobulin (primarily IgA class). These submucosal glands, some of which are serous, others mucous or mixed, have a tubuloacinar structure similar to the salivary glands.

The *deep layer* has a vascular architecture that can be appreciated particularly in the inferior turbinate, the free margin of the middle turbinate and the middle portion of the septum.

The arteries run almost perpendicularly from the deeper to the upper areas of the mucosa where they form a dense subepithelial capillary network; from here, thin-walled venules branch out and join to form the cortical structure of the erectile body. This characteristic structure of the vascular system is typical of the nasal mucosa but is absent in the sinuses.

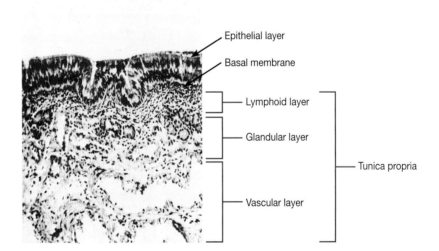

Figure 2.24 Layers of the tunica propria of the nasal mucosa.

Epithelial layer
Basal membrane
Lymphoid layer
Glandular layer
Vascular layer
Tunica propria

Inflammatory Cells

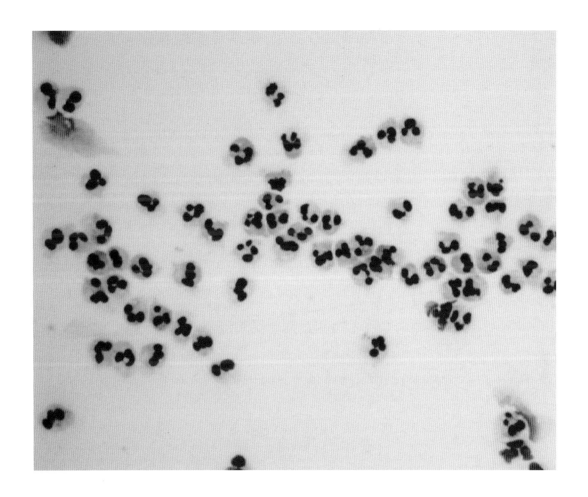

*Learning proceeds by understanding. The forms and colors
cells demonstrate on a smear can be explained by cell
ultrastructure and in this way linked to cell function.*

Marcel Bessis, 1976

Morphology and Classification of Inflammatory Cells

Different types of inflammatory cells may be found in the nasal epithelium, each specific for a certain disease (**Fig. 3.1 a-b**). Identifying these cells and knowing their functions can enhance our understanding of the underlying pathophysiology and can facilitate the selection of appropriate treatment.

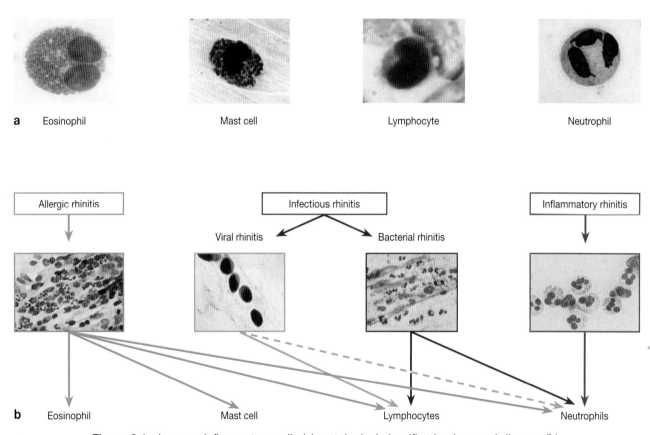

Figure 3.1 Immune-inflammatory cells (**a**); cytological classification by nasal disease (**b**).

NEUTROPHILIC GRANULOCYTES

Neutrophilic granulocytes are round and average 12-14 μm in diameter.

The cell cycle from myeloblast to mature neutrophil spans about 10 days, after which the cell is stored in a peripheral neutrophil pool from which it can quickly be mobilized as required.

The peripheral blood contains about 700 million neutrophils/kg. A neutrophil remains in circulation for approximately 10 hours. It then migrates into the tissues where it phagocytizes and *kills* foreign agents such as microorganisms, toxic substances, foreign material or necrotic products.

Neutrophils have a multilobated (or "poly lobulated") nucleus with a characteristic form, which is why they have been incorrectly termed "polymorphonucleates" (**Fig. 3.2**).

The lobes of the multilobated nucleus are joined together by fine filaments of nuclear material. The nucleus arranges itself in the cytoplasm in a random fashion depending on the way the cell stretches out, often forming an "S", "Y", "Z" or "E" shape visible only on smears.

In vivo observation reveals that the lobes are actually arranged in a circle around the centrosome at the center of the cell. The highly dense chromatin is formed by very dark masses separated by small lighter areas. Nuclear appendages can often be noticed in pathologic states, but are rarely seen in normal conditions.

The degree of polylobulation may be related to the age of the granulocyte. In younger cells, the nucleus appears elongated and folded over, lending it a kidney shape, whereas in older cells it has a neck that separates it into two or more nuclear lobes connected by thin bridges.

According to Arneth's classification (**Fig. 3.3**), six different classes of normal granulocytes may be differentiated. The percentage distribution of each class is listed in **Table 3.1**.

Neutrophilic granules can be found in the cytoplasm mixed with occasional azurophilic granules.

The number of granules varies. Even in normal conditions the quantity of granules may range from few or no granules to an abnormally high number of granules.

Staining intensity varies as well, but such differences are difficult to detect because the granules are so small that they are barely distinguishable under light microscopy. Furthermore, some remnants of

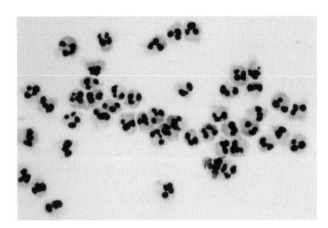

Figure 3.2 Group of neutrophilic granulocytes with characteristic polylobated nucleus.

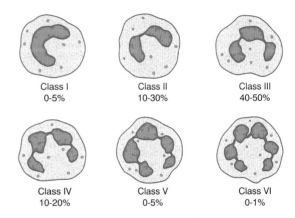

Class I	Class II	Class III
0-5%	10-30%	40-50%

Class IV	Class V	Class VI
10-20%	0-5%	0-1%

Figure 3.3 Arneth count. The percentage distribution of polymorphonuclear neutrophils based on the number of lobes in the nuclei.

primary granulocytes with a certain affinity for azur dye may be mixed among the "neutrophilic" granulocytes. Other causes of variation in staining inten-

Table 3.1 Granulocyte classification according to Arneth stages

Class	No. of nuclear lobes	Distribution (%)
I	Curved or non segmented	0-5
II	2	10-30
III	3	40-50
IV	4	10-20
V	5	0-5
VI	> 5	0-1

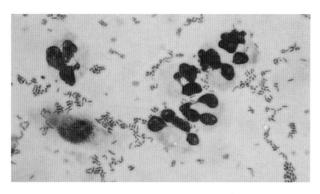

Figure 3.4 Group of neutrophils and numerous inter- and extracellular bacteria (MGG staining; ×1000 with CMF 2.2×).

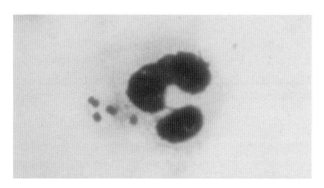

Figure 3.5 Neutrophil summoned by a group of bacteria.

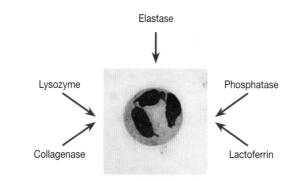

Figure 3.6 Granular enzymes of the neutrophil.

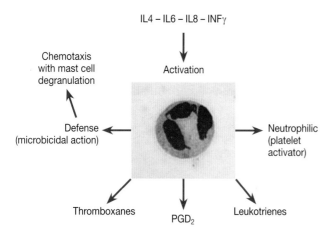

Figure 3.7 Mechanism of action of neutrophil granulocytes.

sity include variations in the staining technique and more frequently differences due to the cell's functional stage.

Examining smears stained with MGG can provide additional information; however, electron microscopy and microcinematography are needed to visualize cell metabolism and phagocytosis.

One of the main functions of neutrophilic granulocytes is ingestion and digestion of germs (**Figs. 3.4, 3.5**). This phenomenon was first described in the early 1900s as microphagia. Granulocytes can phagocytize other cells as well as large non cellular elements such as mineral particles. Hence, they are capable of both microphagia and macrophagia. The general term that would describe both of these processes is *phagocytosis.*

Following phagocytosis, the cytoplasmic granules empty their lytic content into the digestive vacuole, completing their job as killer cells. They can do this thanks to the production of hydrogen peroxide and superoxide, two substances formed in the phagosome from specific oxygenases such as myeloperoxidase (MPO). The hydrolytic enzymes contained in the primary and secondary granules degrade the products that are then digested and eliminated via the exocytotic vesicles (**Figs. 3.6, 3.7**).

In the nasal cytogram of healthy subjects the sporadic occurrence of neutrophils is considered normal, however, an increased number warrants monitoring.

A significant rise in neutrophil count has been observed in recent years, particularly in inhabitants of industrial cities and in those occupationally exposed to inhaled toxic substances or airborne particulates.

The increase in neutrophils is not correlated with the presence of bacteria or fungal spores, or with signs of other cytopathologies, as occurs in infectious disease (**Figs. 3.8, 3.9**). Instead, the granulocytes are activated in these conditions to phagocytize the particulates. Their presence on the mucosa must be transient, otherwise they would release the lytic enzymes they carry.

In our opinion, the increase in non-specific vasomotor rhinitis over the past two decades is due to the release of free radicals which damage the mucosa, resulting in vasomotor dystonia (**Fig. 3.10**).

An elevated neutrophil count also has implications for allergic rhinitis. In seasonal forms of the condition, and particularly in the perennial forms, neutrophils are especially abundant (**Fig. 3.11**). Electron microscopic studies have demonstrated

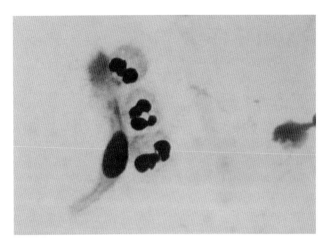

Figure 3.8 Comparison of the size of columnar cells of the respiratory epithelium with that of a neutrophil.

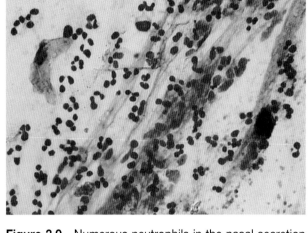

Figure 3.9 Numerous neutrophils in the nasal secretion of a patient with vasomotor rhinitis. No bacterial colonies or infectious agents are present.

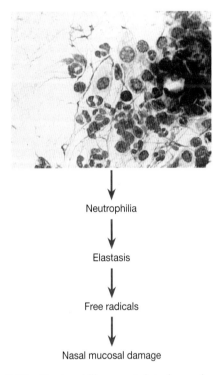

Neutrophilia

↓

Elastasis

↓

Free radicals

↓

Nasal mucosal damage

Figure 3.10 Neutrophilia: postulated mechanism responsible for vasomotor dystonia.

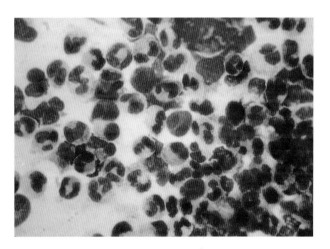

Figure 3.11 Allergic rhinitis. Prevalence of neutrophils on the nasal cytogram (MGG staining; ×1000 with CMF 1.2×).

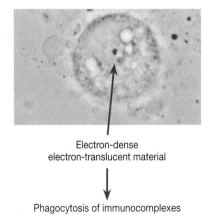

Electron-dense
electron-translucent material

↓

Phagocytosis of immunocomplexes

Figure 3.12 The role of neutrophils in allergic rhinitis.

electron-dense electron-translucent material inside the phagolysosomes.

This material is composed of numerous antigen-antibody immune complexes on the mucosal surface in this disease (**Fig. 3.12**).

EOSINOPHILIC GRANULOCYTES

In 1879 Paul Ehrlich was studying the characteristics of aniline as a dye for staining peripheral blood smears when he noticed that a certain leukocyte with cytoplasmic granules bound avidly to acid dyes. Since a reddish-orange dye called eosin, whose name derives from *Eos* the Greek goddess of the dawn, had a great affinity for the granules in these leukocytes, he coined the term *eosinophil* to describe them (**Fig. 3.13**).

Eosinophils, postmitotic leukocytes of the myeloid cell line, arise in the bone marrow under the effect of differentiation factors IL1, IL3, IL5 and GM-CSF (*granulocyte-macrophage colony stimulating factor*).

After remaining in the bone marrow for about four days, they migrate into the peripheral blood where they have a half-life of less than one day. They then cross the endothelial intercellular junctions by diapedesis and migrate into the tissues. Notably, alterations in vascular permeability can considerably affect the ability of eosinophils to infiltrate the tissues, leading to the pathogenesis of various clinical syndromes.

In healthy individuals, the percentage of eosinophils in the peripheral blood is about 1-6% of the total leukocyte population. But in allergic and non allergic conditions (e.g. parasitosis, chronic inflammations some forms of neoplasia, lung diseases, NARES [*non-allergic rhinitis with eosinophilia syndrome*], etc.) the percentage may rise to over 15-30%.

Morphologically, eosinophils are similar in structure to other granulocytes. Mature eosinophils are slightly larger than neutrophils (9 µm in diameter in fresh preparations and 12-15 µm in smears owing to distension). The nucleus is devoid of a nucleolus, lobulated, but less polymorphous than that of neutrophils, which rarely have less than 2-3 lobes. The chromatin is usually heterochromatic (**Figs. 3.14, 3.15**).

A characteristic feature of eosinophils is that they have primary and secondary intracytoplasmic granules. These granules are normally spherical or lozenge-shaped, range from 0.5 µm to 1.5 µm in diameter, and are larger than those of neutrophils.

Upon examination of the ultrastructure, the granules appear enclosed by a membrane and have a dense matrix, inside which is a variably shaped core consisting of protein macromolecules with a molecular weight of over 1 million Da. These macromolecules are arranged in concentric lamina forming a tubular cavity filled with material similar to that of the granule matrix.

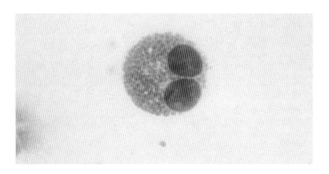

Figure 3.13 Eosinophil. Characteristic bilobated nucleus with acidophil intracytoplasmic granules (MGG staining; ×1000 with CMF 2.2×).

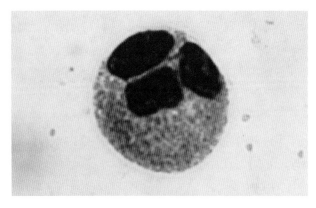

Figure 3.14 Eosinophil with trilobated nucleus (MGG staining; ×1000 with CMF 4.0×).

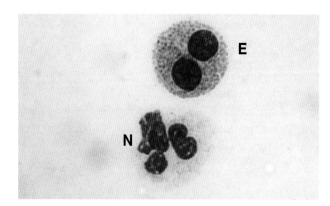

Figure 3.15 Morphologic and staining differences between a neutrophil (N) and an eosinophil (E) (MGG staining; ×1000 with CMF 2.2×).

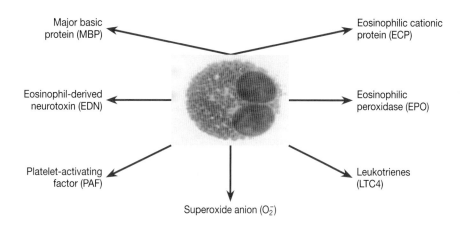

Figure 3.16 Functional components of an eosinophilic granulocyte.

Eosinophils have different functions and occur in different population subsets:
- normodense eosinophils at rest;
- activated normodense eosinophils;
- activated hypodense eosinophils.

The second and particularly the third subset have more membrane receptors and therefore greater functional activity.

Several known functional components include (**Fig. 3.16**):
- membrane components: Charcot-Leyden crystal (CLC) protein exhibiting lysophospholipid activity. Since this phospholipid is easily crystallized, it is often found in the stools of bronchial asthma patients;
- granular components: major basic protein (MBP), eosinophilic cationic protein (ECP), eosinophilic protein X (EPX), eosinophilic peroxidase (EPO);
- non granular components:
  - enzymes (arylsulfatase A, phospholipase D, histaminase, collagenase, phosphatase acids) that play an important role in the self-regulation of allergic inflammatory response;
  - metabolites of arachidonic acid (LTC4, HETE, PGD_2, PGE_1) which are new mediators, some of which have bronchoconstrictor action, and numerous cytokines (IL2, IL6, IL8, IL16),

TNFα, as well as differentiation factors (including IL3, IL5, GM-CSF), that augment eosinophil chemotaxis (**Fig. 3.17**).

Recent studies have shown the particular function of major basic protein (MBP); this can attack the desmosomal intercellular junctions, exposing the mucosa of the nasal cavity and the respiratory tract to chemical, physical and infectious agents (**Fig. 3.18**). This process is prominent in some forms of asthma. Cells undergoing intercellular scission form so-called "Creola bodies", first found in a subject who died of an acute asthma attack (**Fig. 3.19**).

The exact lifespan of eosinophils has not yet been established but is thought to be from two to five days depending on the type of tissue.

The way eosinophils disappear is unknown. Some are phagocytized, as demonstrated by the finding of typical granules inside the phagosomes of macrophages; others, as occurs with neutrophils, are eliminated via the gut and lungs.

A morphologic-diagnostic consideration to be kept in mind when searching for eosinophils is that in some cases the cells do not demonstrate their typical characteristics (bilobed cell with eosinophilic granules), but rather present a single trilobed nucleus (**Fig. 3.20**).

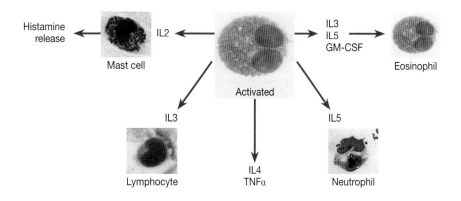

Figure 3.17 Non granular components of an eosinophilic granulocyte.

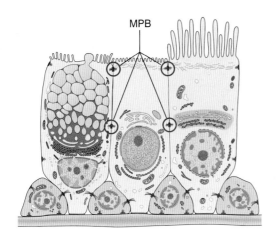

Figure 3.18 Sites of major basic protein (MBP) lysis in the desmosomal junctions.

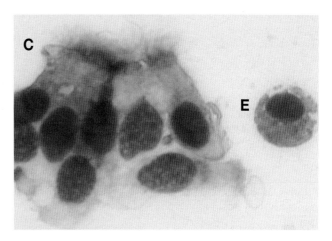

Figure 3.19 Group of respiratory mucosal cells (C); Creola body in a patient with allergic rhinitis and asthma. Eosinophil (E) (MGG staining; ×1000 with CMF 1.2×).

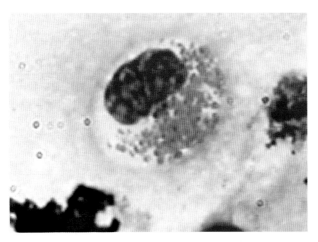

Figure 3.20 Eosinophil with prominent intracytoplasmic granules; the nucleus appears as a single body.

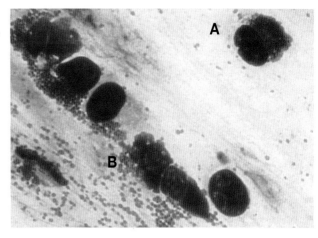

Figure 3.21 Eosinophils in partial (A) and complete degranulation (B) (MGG staining; ×1000 with CMF 1.2×).

In acute phase allergic rhinitis, especially pollen-induced forms, eosinophils may not appear intact but may instead exhibit partial or complete degranulation (**Fig. 3.21**). Only by identifying numerous dispersed granules with typical eosinophilic color can the cytologist establish a correct diagnosis (**Fig. 3.22**).

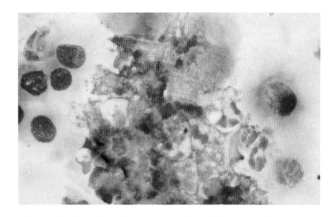

Figure 3.22 Nasal cytology in which no cellular elements are recognizable; however, the typical staining features of the granules suggest a diagnosis of massive eosinophil degranulation with cell degradation in a patient with acute phase allergic rhinitis (MGG staining; ×1000).

MAST CELLS

In mammals, mast cells are widely distributed throughout the body, on the mucosal and serous surfaces, in lymphoid and connective tissues, as well as associated with nervous, vascular and neoplastic tissues (**Figs. 3.23-3.25**).

Their nearly ubiquitous distribution distinguishes them from basophils which invade the tissues only during inflammatory events.

In the bronchial and nasal mucosa, mast cells are located at the interface with the external environment, making them front-line cells in the body's defense against inhaled allergens. This has been demonstrated by the finding of mast cell-induced mediators in nasal lavage liquid after allergen challenge testing.

Mast cell precursors arise in the bone marrow before migrating into the peripheral blood and then into the tissues where they mature under the effect of certain cytokines. Studies on rodents suggest that in the bone marrow mast cell precursor replication and recruitment are stimulated by IL4 and IgE complexes.

The histologic features of mast cells and basophils have fascinated scientists since the time of Ehrlich's experiments in the 1870s in which he showed that these cells stained metachromatically with certain dyes. Today, dyes like toluidine blue are still routinely used to stain mast cells and basophils.

However, the metachromatic histochemical reaction in which the basic dye interacts with the acid proteoglycans in mast cells and basophils has definite drawbacks since it does not permit mast cells to

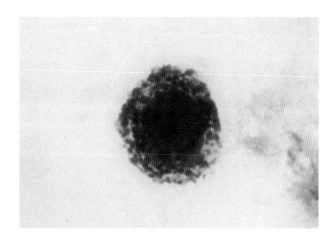

Figure 3.23 Mast cell. The nucleus appears roughly kidney-shaped, partly covered by basophilic granules. The intracytoplasmic granules are larger than the eosinophilic granules (MGG staining; ×1000 with CMF 4×).

be distinguished from basophils, which are differentiated according to other morphologic characteristics. Moreover, the staining conditions need to be meticulously controlled, and even then true metachromasia may be difficult to interpret, leading to errors in calculating the mast cell count.

Mast cells and basophils are characterized by membrane-bound receptors with a high affinity for IgE. Immunologic stimulation of mast cells causes exocytosis of granule-associated preformed mediators and the *de novo* synthesis of eicosanoids (derived from arachidonic acid metabolism) (**Fig. 3.26**).

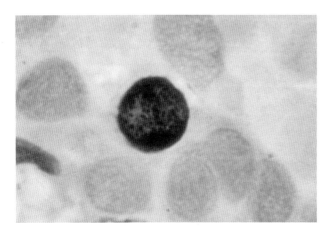

Figure 3.24 Mast cell in a nasal secretion. Characteristic metachromatic staining of the granules which nearly cover the nucleus (MGG staining; ×1000 with CMF 1.4×).

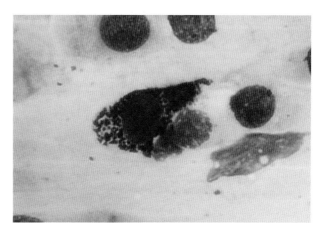

Figure 3.25 Degranulating mast cell (MGG staining; ×1000 with CMF 1.4×).

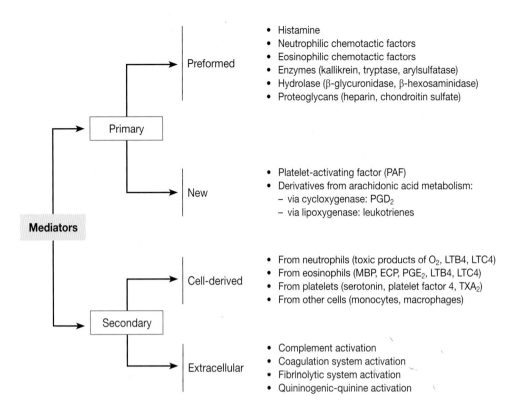

- Preformed
  - Histamine
  - Neutrophilic chemotactic factors
  - Eosinophilic chemotactic factors
  - Enzymes (kallikrein, tryptase, arylsulfatase)
  - Hydrolase (β-glycuronidase, β-hexosaminidase)
  - Proteoglycans (heparin, chondroitin sulfate)

- New
  - Platelet-activating factor (PAF)
  - Derivatives from arachidonic acid metabolism:
    - via cycloxygenase: PGD_2
    - via lipoxygenase: leukotrienes

- Cell-derived
  - From neutrophils (toxic products of O_2, LTB4, LTC4)
  - From eosinophils (MBP, ECP, PGE_2, LTB4, LTC4)
  - From platelets (serotonin, platelet factor 4, TXA_2)
  - From other cells (monocytes, macrophages)

- Extracellular
  - Complement activation
  - Coagulation system activation
  - Fibrinolytic system activation
  - Quininogenic-quinine activation

Figure 3.26 Mast cell mediators.

Mast cells have long been thought to play an important role in the acute phase of allergic inflammation. They are also believed to be responsible for the initial events of chronic allergic inflammation. Specifically, histamine, tryptase, PGD_2 and LTC4 derived from mast cells are involved in the immediate response to allergen provocation (**Figs. 3.27, 3.28**).

In the nasal cavity, mast cell mediators induce rhinorrhea, nasal obstruction and sneezing by acting on the microvessels and sensory nerve endings (**Fig. 3.29**).

The concomitant production of LTC4, PGD_2, chemotactic factors and cytokines initiates leukocyte adhesion, migration and priming (**Figs. 3.30-3.32**).

On reaching the site of allergenic stimulation, these migrating cells interact with the allergen. This interaction or the elevated local concentration of cytokines induces mediator release. IL4 also stimulates prolonged *de novo* synthesis of IL3, IL4, IL5, IL10 and GM-CSF by Th2 (T helper 2) lymphocytes, which work mainly to induce the production of IgE

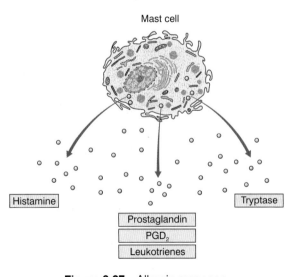

Figure 3.27 Allergic response.

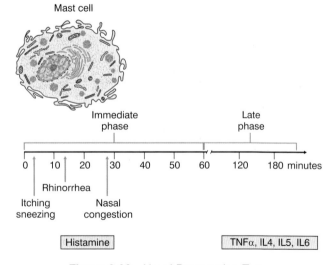

Figure 3.28 Nasal Provocation Test.

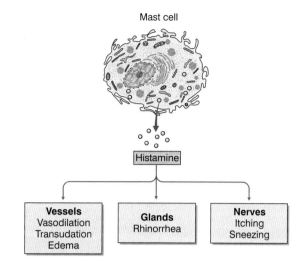

Figure 3.29 Allergic response.

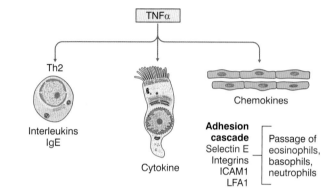

Figure 3.30 Adhesion activities.

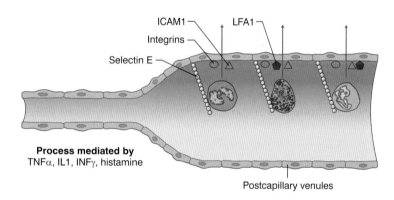

Figure 3.31 Leukocyte migration.

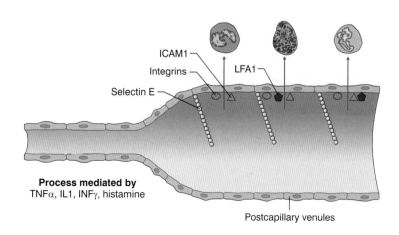

Figure 3.32 Leukocyte priming.

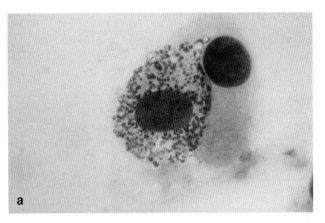

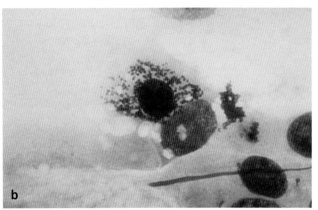

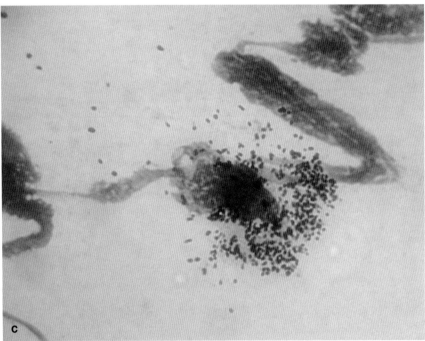

Figure 3.33 a-c Phases of mast cell degranulation (MGG staining; ×1000 with CMF 1.4× (**a-b**) and 4.0× (**c**).

by B lymphocytes and to maintain the chronic allergic inflammatory response.

In brief, mast cells may be considered one of the main cell types responsible for the induction of the immediate allergenic response and chronic allergic inflammation, where the end phase consists of massive degranulation and release of primary and secondary chemical mediators (**Figs. 3.24, 3.26, 3.33**).

LYMPHOCYTES

Lymphocytes are the circulating components responsible for cellular and humoral immunity (**Figs. 3.34-3.36**). During the first years of life, they account for 30-70% of white blood cells in the peripheral blood and 10-30% of bone marrow cells. Based on the type of immune response they initiate, they may be classified as:

- T lymphocytes;
- B lymphocytes;
- non T-non B lymphocytes, so-called null lymphocytes.

In the inactivated state, the three lymphocyte subpopulations cannot be differentiated from one another. To do this, it is necessary to utilize typing of the membrane antigens normally present on the cytoplasmic membrane.

Morphologic Classes of Lymphocytes

Morphologically, lymphocytes can be differentiated as:

- small lymphocytes;
- large lymphocytes;
- activated lymphocytes.

Small Lymphocytes

T and B lymphocytes are most often small lymphocytes. They have a round nucleus and a thin rim of agranular cytoplasm. The nuclear chromatin is dense and stains intensely. Usually, they display rounded borders or sometimes cytoplasmic protrusions. The cytoplasm stains blue, with shades pale to intense in color. Their diameter ranges from 7 μm to 10 μm.

These cells are quiescent, but are ready to react on stimulation by an external agent.

Large Lymphocytes

Large lymphocytes account for 5-10% of circulating lymphocytes. The diameter of the larger cells is about two to three times that of small lymphocytes. Their form, staining and nuclear chromatin

structure are similar to those of small lymphocytes. The nucleoli are not normally visible. The extensive cytoplasm has a basophilic tinge (**Fig. 3.37**).

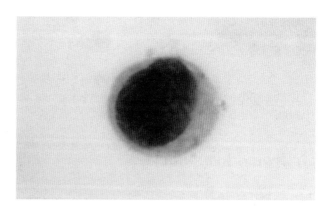

Figure 3.34 Lymphocyte.

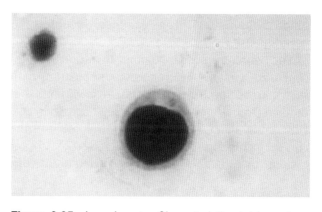

Figure 3.35 Lymphocyte. Characteristic staining of cytoplasm (blue sky). The small translucent area inside is the centrosome.

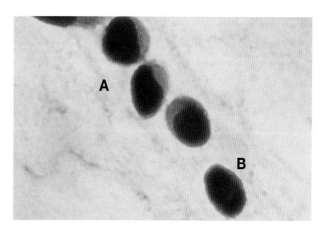

Figure 3.36 Group of lymphocytes (A); eosinophil (B).

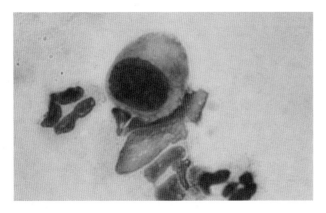

Figure 3.37 Large lymphocyte. The nucleoli are not usually visible. Extensive cytoplasm with a basophilic tinge (MGG staining; ×1000 with CMF 2.2×).

Killer and natural killer T lymphocytes make up the bulk of this class.

Activated Lymphocytes

Larger than the preceding two classes, these lymphocytes have a round, indented or lobulated nucleus, the chromatin is more scattered and the nucleoli are sometimes visible. The extensive basophilic cytoplasm displays granules, vacuoles and pseudopods.

The lymphocytes that respond to antigen stimuli constitute a highly heterogeneous population with such a broad spectrum of morphologic variants that they are sometimes termed or called atypical cells. Differential diagnosis is based on evaluation of the clinical picture.

Some investigators believe that, owing to the con-

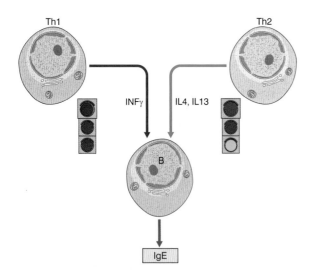

Figure 3.38 Th2 lymphocytes can release cytokines, including IL4, which is responsible for IgE oriented isotype switching.

siderable polymorphism characterizing these cells, they should be called "lymphocytic variants" rather than "activated and/or atypical lymphocytes". Another reason to do this is because the morphologic changes they undergo in response to antigens are, from an immunologic standpoint, typical of normally functioning cells.

Functional Classes of Lymphocytes

Depending on where they reside, lymphocytes can act as killers (T lymphocytes) or as mediators (B lymphocytes) that induce the release of antibodies.

T Lymphocytes

Thymus-derived lymphocytes (T lymphocytes) induce cell-mediated sensitivity. They act directly on the *non-self* invader, inhibiting its growth and killing its extraneous elements. They cooperate with other immune system cells to defend the host organism against viral and bacterial infection.

T lymphocytes play a key role in the development and maintenance of allergic conditions and T helper (Th) lymphocytes are divided into subsets according to function and the type of cytokine they produce.

At least three different T lymphocyte subpopulations have been described so far:
- Th1 lymphocytes produce IL2, interferon (IFN) and tumor necrosis factor (TNF);
- Th2 lymphocytes produce IL4, IL5 and IL13;
- Th0 lymphocytes produce the same classes of interleukins as both Th1 and Th2 lymphocytes.

B Lymphocytes

Some stem cells have been shown to migrate from the blood into *bursa-like organs* (so-called because they resemble the bursa of Fabricius in birds), where they come into contact with epithelial cells. The lymphocytes that develop in these structures are termed B lymphocytes and are responsible for humoral immunity. When stimulated by antigens, some respond by transforming into cells with a basophilic cytoplasm and blastoid chromatin features. Within a couple of days, these cells then transform into active plasma cells.

Lymphocyte activity is a major contributing factor in the pathogenesis of allergic rhinitis (**Figs. 3.38, 3.39**). In the pathogenesis of the allergic response, the prevalence of Th2 lymphocytes plays a

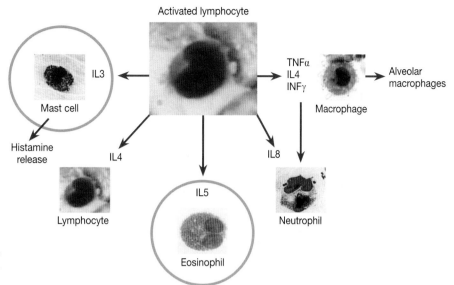

Figure 3.39 Lymphocytes are among the primary elements of allergic inflammation.

key part because of their ability to release cytokines, specifically IL4, which is chiefly responsible for IgE isotype switching. In the presence of IL4, T lympho- cytes present the antigen to B lymphocytes which, on stimulation by IL2 and IL6, transform into plasma cells that synthesize specific IgE.

PLASMA CELLS

Plasma cells account for about 1% of nuclear cells in healthy bone marrow and measure 15-25 μm in diameter. On a rhinocytogram, they appear rounded or oval, with smooth or slightly irregular borders. The oval nucleus is usually located at one pole of the cytoplasm; its longest diameter is perpendicular to that of the cytoplasm.

The chromatin has a characteristic tortoiseshell or wheel-like appearance since the chromocenters are distributed in large clumps (about 7-9) roughly polygonal in shape (**Fig. 3.40**).

The cytoplasm exhibits intense basophilia, its sea blue color rendering it immediately recognizable. The centrosome is colorless or stains slightly. Many plasma cells contain one or more vacuoles, whereas phagocytic particles are absent.

Intracytoplasmic accumulations of immunoglobulins can sometimes produce variations in the form and staining features of plasma cells, making it hard to identify them by morphologic criteria alone.

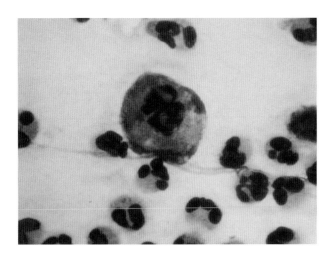

Figure 3.40 Plasma cell. Typical features are the wheel-like appearance of the nuclear chromatin and basophilic cytoplasm (MGG staining; ×1000 with CMF 1.2×).

MACROPHAGES

Arising from monocytic stem cells in the bone marrow, macrophages pass into the bloodstream from where they migrate into the tissues where they develop and mature. Macrophages have a relatively long lifespan of several months.

In healthy tissues, they are generally at rest but can be activated to perform numerous functions. During inflammatory events, circulating monocytes are recruited to the tissues. This recruitment may be massive in conditions of chronic inflammation, including those caused by microorganisms that neutrophils cannot readily digest, so-called intracellular bacteria.

Macrophages are round in shape, with a kidney-shaped nucleus and extensive cytoplasm where digestive vacuoles containing cell or bacterial debris can be found (**Figs. 3.41-3.46**).

All macrophages, whether residing in connective tissue interspaces of the airways or elsewhere, or arising from monocytes and recruited to the site of inflammatory response, perform a variety of functions. During inflammatory processes, they carry out at least four functions:

- Phagocytic function. Macrophages contain a host of digestive enzymes similar to those of neutrophils, as well as the NADPH oxidase, an enzyme complex almost identical to that of neutrophils. Their microbicidal activity is exerted inside the phagocytic vacuole and is strongest when the cell is activated by cytokines such as interferon gamma (IFNγ).
- Antigen processing. Macrophages can process antigens and microorganisms, partially digesting them to produce polypeptides that are then associated with molecules coded by the major histocompatibility complex (i.e. HLA, the *human leucocyte antigen complex*). Recognition of these complexes (processed antigens associated with HLA molecules expressed on the macrophage surface) by T lymphocytes is a key step in the activation of the immune response.
- Ecologic function. Macrophages are primarily responsible for ridding the alveolar spaces of inhaled microorganisms and particles. It is thought that a single macrophage can clean up at least

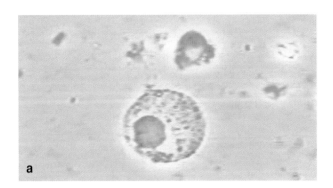

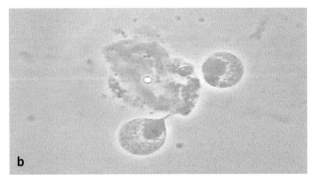

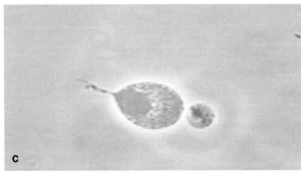

Figure 3.42 Macrophage (phase-contrast microscopy). Phases of phagocytosis. Macrophage containing numerous bacteria (**a**); macrophage during phagocytosis: distinct filopodium englobing a bacterium (**b**); expulsion of debris and dead bacteria from the exocytotic vesicle (**c**).

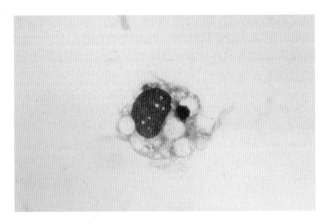

Figura 3.41 Macrophage (MGG staining; ×1000 with CMF 1.2×).

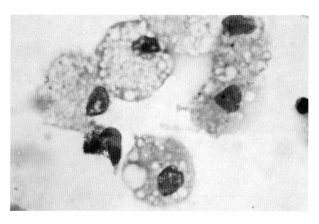

Figure 3.43 Induced expectorate. Numerous macrophages present in the lung. Characteristically, these macrophages have an oval nucleus and extensive cytoplasm filled with numerous digestive vacuoles (MGG staining; ×1000 with CMF 1.2×).

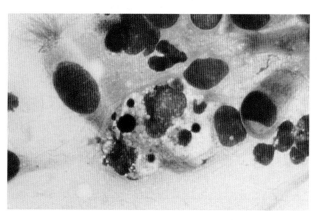

Figure 3.44 Macrophage. The cytoplasm contains corpuscles and cell debris resulting from phagocytosis (MGG staining; ×1000 with CMF 1.2×).

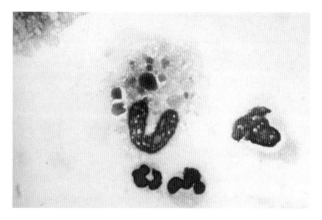

Figure 3.45 Macrophage. The kidney-shaped nucleus has a prominent nucleolus. The cytoplasm is filled with products of phagocytosis (cell debris, bacteria, etc.) (MGG staining; ×1000 with CMF 1.2×).

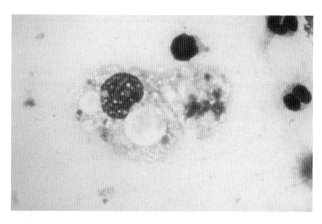

Figure 3.46 Macrophage. The cytoplasm is filled with products of phagocytosis (cell debris, bacteria, vacuoles, etc.) and large digestive vacuoles (MGG staining; ×1000).

three alveoli. But they are also involved in cleaning up the tissues after an inflammatory event since they can recognize and phagocytize cell debris and dead cells, including neutrophils and neutral fragments.

• Secretory function. Macrophagic secretion influences the course of inflammation by synthesizing and releasing numerous molecules, including cytokines IL1, IL8, TNFα, and GM-CSF.

Sometimes, during the Masters courses, and the students' introduction to microscopic analysis, they have found it difficult to visualize macrophages in the microscopic preparations at their disposal. This difficulty is due to the fact that the nasal macrophage population is significantly smaller than the alveolar macrophage population, due to the two different types of defense systems characterizing these two respiratory areas. In the presence of a system of mucociliary *clearance* (nasal cavity and bronchi), the macrophage population is smaller. This situation is reversed at the alveolar level where macrophages are the most common cells found (**Fig. 3.43**).

Inflammatory Agents

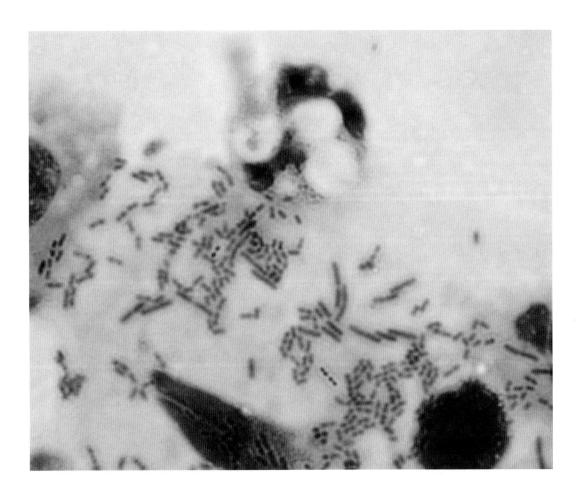

*I wish to thank Professor Maria Teresa Montagna,
Institute of Hygiene, University of Bari,
for her useful suggestions in writing this chapter.
Her help, in clarifyng the subject matter, was essential.*

Pathogenic Microorganisms: Bacteria, Fungi and Viruses

At the end of the 1600s, Antoni van Leeuwenhoek, inventor of the first microscope, managed to observe the shape and life of tiny creatures, invisible to the naked eye, and produced interesting and important drawings of them. For his description of these miniscule living beings, which exist below the limits of the human eye, Leeuwenhoek may be regarded as the father of bacterioscopy.

I decided to include this chapter on pathogens because anyone involved in nasal cytology is bound to become something of a microbiologist, and also because "the more you know, the more you see". Being equipped with a "basic" knowledge of microbiology allows the cytologist not only to understand the patient better, from the clinical perspective, but also to be open to new fields of research and ready to make new scientific contributions. Contributions that nasal cytology has made to microbiology in recent years include the description of the *infectious spot*, which is the morphologic-chromatic expression of biofilm, and of the cell changes in the nasal mucosa induced by herpes viruses.

BACTERIA

Bacteria are normal inhabitants of the nasal cavity and sinuses, which are never completely sterile, and potentially pathogenic bacteria can colonize the nasal vestibule and nasopharynx of healthy individuals (**Fig. 4.1**).

Viral infections can modify the mucociliary clearance mechanism, thereby facilitating overgrowth of the normal nasal-sinus flora.

Microorganisms isolated from the nasal cavity and nasopharynx of healthy adults include:

- *Staphylococcus epidermidis* and *Micrococcus*;
- *Staphylococcus aureus*;
- *Streptococcus pneumoniae*;
- *Streptococcus pyogenes*;
- Diphtheroids;
- *Haemophilus influenzae*;
- Moraxella;
- Neisseria;
- Gram-negative bacteria.

Most bacteria have staining and morphologic features that can be seen under a light microscope. By isolating them on an appropriate culture medium, they can be more accurately identified making it possible to institute targeted therapy rather than empirical treatments, as often occurs.

Staphylococcus

Staphylococci are round (cocci), Gram-positive, asporigenic, strictly aerobic (rarely anaerobic), non motile bacteria.

The name *Staphylococcus* derives from the random aggregation of cell clusters of various sizes (**Fig.**

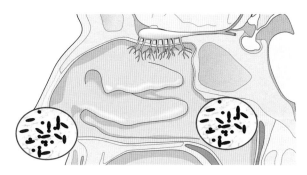

Figure 4.1 When there is an intact mucociliary clearance system bacteria generally colonize the nasal vestibule and nasopharynx.

4.2 a-b), but cells may also be found singly, in pairs or tetrads.

These clusters possess many cell components and produce a wide variety of extracellular substances such as enzymes and toxins, a capability which gives them varying levels of pathogenicity. Many of these cell components and extracellular substances are exclusive to *Staphylococcus aureus*, the only species pathogenic for humans. Other species (*S. epidermidis*, *S. saprophyticus*, *S. hominis*, *S. auricularis*, etc.) are mostly commensals and are therefore considered opportunistic pathogens.

The genus *Staphylococcus* differs from that of *Micrococcus* in that the latter is unable to ferment glucose in anaerobiosis.

Streptococcus

Streptococci are Gram-positive, asporogenic, facultative aerobic, but sometimes strictly anaerobic,

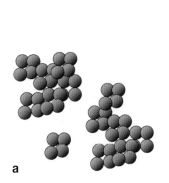
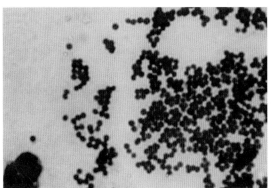

Figure 4.2 Schematic diagram of staphylococci (**a**). Groups of staphylococci isolated from nasal secretion (MGG staining; ×1000 with CMF 2×; **b**).

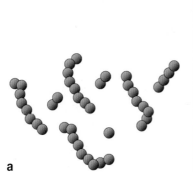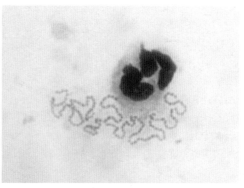

a

b

Figure 4.3 Schematic diagram of streptococci (**a**). Group of streptococci isolated from nasal secretion (MGG staining; ×1000) (**b**).

non motile cocci. They are usually arranged in long chains of oval or spherical cells (**Fig. 4.3 a-b**), rarely occurring singly or in pairs.

Chain length, no longer considered an index of their virulence, depends on the composition of the culture medium – longer chains form in a liquid medium – and varies according to the species or isolated strain.

The most important species from a clinical point of view belong to group A (*Streptococcus pyogenes*), which produces beta-hemolysis on blood agar.

Streptococcus Pneumoniae

Pneumococci are Gram-positive, capsulated diplococci having a characteristic lancet or ovoid shape (**Fig. 4.4 a-b**). In liquid medium they frequently aggregate in short chains.

On cell lysis, they release toxins (pneumolysin) and proinflammatory cell wall products.

In 30-70% of cases, they can be isolated from the nasopharynx of healthy individuals; in weakened subjects they can cause severe pneumonia, otitis media, sinusitis, meningitis, pericarditis and septicemia.

Diphtheroids

Diphtheroids comprise species of Gram-positive bacilli belonging to the genus *Corynebacterium* but differing from *Corynebacterium diphtheriae*. These pleomorphic microbes have metachromatic granules and are often enlarged at one end of the cell body, giving them a club-shaped appearance, whence their name. Microscopically, they appear arranged in parallel rows (i.e. palisade arrangement) or joined at one end ("finger" or "Chinese letter" arrangement) (**Fig. 4.5 a-b**).

Widespread in nature, occurring both in the environment (soil and water) and on human skin and mucosa, they were once considered solely commensal bacteria but are now attributed a pathogenic role, particularly in immunocompromised subjects.

Haemophilus

The haemophilus bacteria are Gram-negative, pleomorphic, facultative aerobic, non motile rods. They are common commensal organisms in the upper respiratory tract (**Fig. 4.6 a-b**).

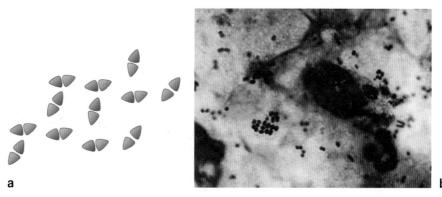

a

b

Figure 4.4 Schematic diagram of pneumococci (**a**). Groups of pneumococci isolated from nasal secretion. In the upper part of the microscopic field it is possible to see a typically cyan-colored "infectious spot" (MGG staining; ×1000 with CMF 1.6×) (**b**).

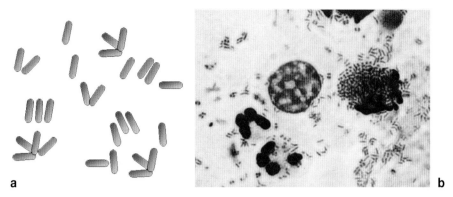

Figure 4.5 Schematic diagram of diphtheroids (**a**). Typical "finger" or palisade arrangement (**b**; MGG staining; ×1000 with CMF 1.4×).

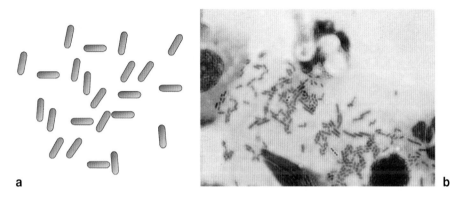

Figure 4.6 Schematic diagram of haemophilus bacteria (**a**). Group of haemophilus bacteria isolated from nasal secretion (**b**; MGG staining; ×1000 with CMF 2.2×).

Haemophilus bacteria colonize the nasopharynx of about 80% of infants within the first year of life and 100% of children and adolescents, before declining in adults.

Haemophilus influenzae, once thought to be responsible for causing influenza, is by far the species best known in human diseases. Its potential pathogenicity is correlated with the presence of a capsule. The pathogenic role of *Haemophilus parainfluenzae* has recently been reviewed.

Moraxella

Moraxella bacteria are Gram-negative, intracellular diplococci (rarely coccobacilli) that grow in conditions of microaerophilia or anaerobiosis (**Fig. 4.7 a-b**). They generally occur in the upper airways of healthy individuals.

The best known species are *M. catarrhalis*, formerly called *Neisseria catarrhalis* and *Branhamella catarrhalis*. They are often the cause of otitis media and sinusitis in children.

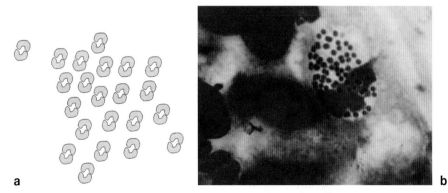

Figure 4.7 Schematic diagram of moraxella bacteria (**a**). Intracellular moraxella bacteria in nasal secretion (**b**; MGG staining; ×1000 with CMF 2.4×).

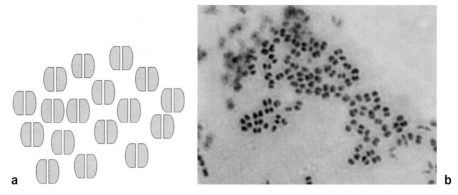

Figure 4.8 Schematic diagram of Neisseria bacteria (**a**). Group of Neisseria isolated from nasal secretion (**b**; MGG staining; ×1000 with CMF 2×).

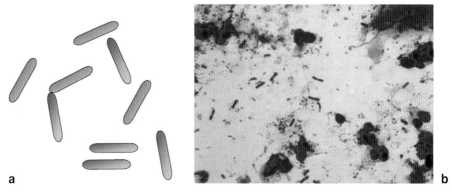

Figure 4.9 Schematic diagram of Pseudomonas (**a**); Pseudomonas isolated from nasal secretion (**b**; MGG staining; ×1000 with CMF 1.4×).

Neisseria

Neisseria are Gram-negative strictly aerobic, non motile diplococci with flattened adjacent sides. In microscopic preparations they resemble coffee beans (**Fig. 4.8**). The different species cannot be differentiated on the basis of morphology.

Their elective site is the oropharyngeal mucosa but they can also be found in the nasal cavity.

Except for *Neisseria gonorrheae* and *Neisseria meningitidis*, which cause gonorrhea and meningococcal meningitis, respectively, other *Neisseria* species are considered commensal bacteria.

Pseudomonas

The Pseudomonas bacteria are Gram-negative, strictly aerobic, motile polar flagellate non fermentative rods (**Fig. 4.9 a-b**).

Pseudomonas species are generally considered opportunistic pathogens. They are particularly significant in hospital-acquired infections; *P. aeruginosa* causes pneumonia, especially in patients with cystic fibrosis, and severe complications (cystitis, sepsis) in immunocompromised patients.

FUNGI

Fungi, or mycetes, are eukaryotic microorganisms that are widely present in the environment and in decomposing organic material. They thrive as saprophytes and opportunistic pathogens in humans and animals. They have a vegetative body (*thallus*) and present a well-defined cell wall devoid of peptidoglycans and theicoic acids, but rich in chitin, glucans, mannans, lipids and glycoproteins. The three-layered cytoplasmic membrane is rich in ergosterol, enclosing a true nucleus containing a nucleolus, mitochondria, vacuoles, ribosomes and other organelles.

Fungi are devoid of chlorophyll; they reproduce by dispersal of sexual or asexual spores (**Fig. 4.10**).

It is impossible to determine how many different types of fungi occur in nature. It is estimated that there are over 100,000 species, very few of which are pathogenic for humans.

Because of their vegetative body, fungi are classified as *yeasts*, which are unicellular organisms that multiply by budding (**Fig. 4.11 a-b, 4.12, 4.13, 4.14**), and multicellular molds with a filamentous mycelium composed of long filaments, or *hyphae*.

Hyphae can be subdivided into cells by septa (*septate hyphae*) (**Fig. 4.13**) or they may be non septate. Depending on the species, septate hyphae cells have one or more nuclei.

The different segments or portions of the mycelium separated by a septum in the same hypha intercommunicate by protoplasmic appendages that allow the nucleus to migrate back and forth.

Nearly all fungi reproduce by germination of a spore (1 μm in diameter) under appropriate conditions of humidity and temperature.

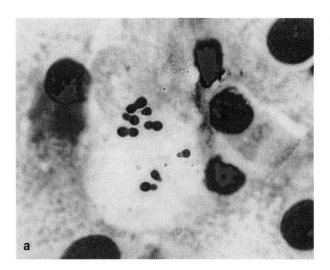

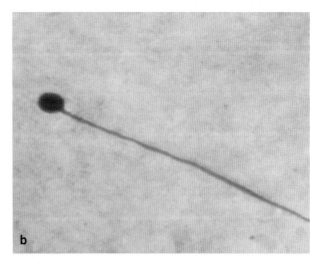

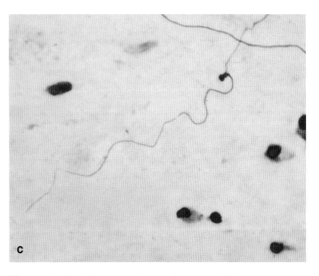

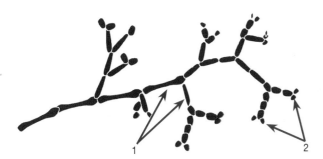

Figure 4.10 The body or thallus of fungi consists of two distinct parts: the vegetative part (1) involved in growth and food intake and the reproductive part (2) involved in propagation and dispersal of the species.

Figure 4.11 Gemmated yeast spores (**a**); zygomycete (**b**); filamentous mycelium (**c**). This is the best image resolution that can be achieved with the magnifying power of today's microscopes (MGG staining; ×1000).

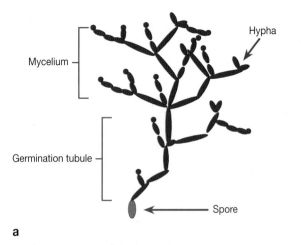

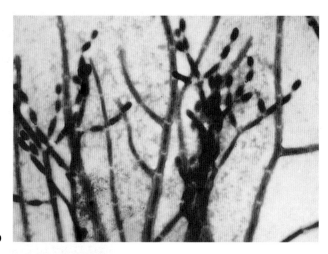

a

b

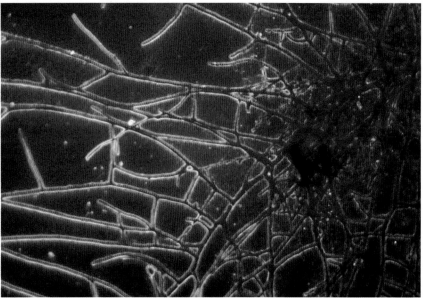

Figure 4.12 Schematic diagram of a fungus (**a**); cytologic preparation (MGG staining; ×1000) (**b**); cytologic sample (dark field microscopy; ×1000 with CMF 2×) (**c**).

c

Germination produces one or more filaments, called *germination tubules* or *promycelia*, into which one or more nuclei and most of the spore protoplasm migrate (**Fig. 4.12 a-c**).

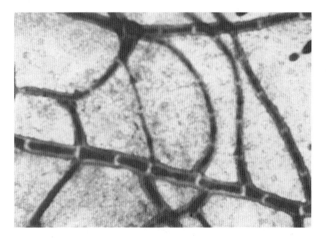

Figure 4.13 Septate hyphae (MGG staining; ×1000).

The study of fungal morphology and staining features is fundamental for taxonomic classification of an isolated species.

An accurate description of a fungal colony should always include the macro- and microscopic features of the mycelium, the hyphae, whether or not septate, modes of branching, development and reproductive body (sporophore, conidiophore, sporangiophore, etc.).

To appreciate fungal morphology, a fresh preparation of fungi is examined under phase-contrast microscopy (**Fig. 4.14 a-c**). Sometimes, however, preparation set-up using a cover glass has the drawback of altering the connections between the various parts (blastospores, conidia, fruit bodies, etc.). Observation should focus on the morphology of the vegetative and reproductive bodies.

On examination of sexual (*asci* and *ascospores*) and asexual (*conidial*) spores, the shape, average size and modes of insertion should be accurately de-

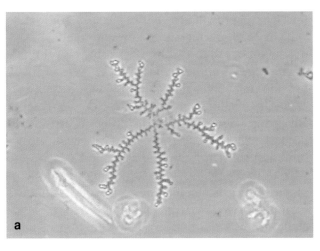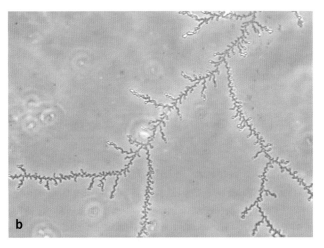

Figure 4.14 Fungal hyphae (phase-contrast microscopy). Initial (**a**) and advanced (**b**) arborizations.

scribed. A full description of morphologic features can aid in systematically classifying the type of fungus in question.

The characteristics of the main genera of fungi responsible for opportunistic fungal infections are described below.

Aspergillus

This is probably the genus with the most species (about 200), about ten of which cause human diseases. They reproduce asexually but some species can also reproduce sexually.

Characterized mainly by septate hyphae, *Aspergillus fungi* are composed of a mycelium that produces a variety of enzymes very like that of other filamentous fungi. Some species can process toxic substances (*mycotoxins*) in which carcinogenic activity has been demonstrated.

The conidia are produced in chains by particular structures (*phialides*) attached either directly to the vesicle or via a supporting cell, the *metula*, (spherical, hemispherical or club-shaped). Frequently flask-shaped, the phialides cover the vesicle surface entirely or partly. These formations constitute the end part of a hypha called a *conidiophore*. The microscopic features of conidiophores (length, diameter, smooth or spiny surface, color, etc.) together with the attributes of the vesicle and the conidia permit the identification of different species (**Fig. 4.15**).

The best known are:
- *A. candidus*;
- *A. clavatus*;
- *A. flavus*;
- *A. fumigatus*;

- *A. glaucus*;
- *A. nidulans*;
- *A. niger*;
- *A. ochraceus*;
- *A. terreus*;
- *A. versicolor*.

The most common clinical manifestations are:
- allergic aspergillosis;
- invasive aspergillosis in immunocompromised patients;
- infections of the paranasal sinuses, the central nervous system, the gastrointestinal tract;
- otomycosis;
- osteomyelitis.

Organ transplant recipients, especially liver transplant patients, are at high risk of this infection.

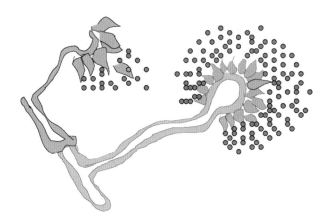

Figure 4.15 Schematic diagram of *Aspergillus*.

Penicillium

Of the many species of *Penicillium*, *P. marneffei* is the only one recognized as being pathogenic for humans and animals.

Penicillium grows rapidly. The colonies are initially white and then turn gray green; but the reverse can also occur, with dark changing to white depending on the species.

The hyphae are septate; the philiades are organized in brush-like clusters at the tips of the conidiophores and attached to the metulae; the conidia are visualized as unbranching chains at the tips of the philiades (**Fig. 4.16**).

When *Penicillium* is isolated from biologic material, a diagnosis of penicillosis can be confirmed only histologically.

Zygomycetes

The fungi belonging to the class of Zygomycetes share certain morphologic features:
- the hyphae are devoid of septae and vary greatly in diameter (5-20 μm);
- the asexual spores are produced inside vesicles attached to a hyphae (*sporangiophore*);
- in sexual reproduction, the male and female elements can be found on the same or different hyphae (**Fig. 4.17**).

Infectious Spot, the Morphologic-Chromatic Expression of Biofilm

For a long time in the history of microbiology, microorganisms were regarded as planktonic organisms, i.e. cells suspended and classified according to their type of growth in a culture medium. And yet, as early as 1600, Anton van Leeuwenhoek, after scraping the surface of teeth, observed, using his primitive microscope, "*animaluculae*"; these were actually nothing other than microbial colonies. It took several years of clinical studies and the development of advanced diagnostic tools in order to arrive at a deeper understanding of the chemical-genetic-structural aspects of these bacterial groups, which were later termed *biofilms*. Indeed, through ultramicroscopic studies using different microscopy techniques (scanning electron, transmission, confocal, laser, etc.), we now know that 15% of biofilm is made up of bacterial and /or fungal colonies, which are surrounded by an organic matrix (constituting the other 85%), which these colonies produce and whose skeleton is made up of exopolysaccharides (EPS). The quantity of EPS varies, depending on the organism, and the amount of EPS increases with the increasing age of the biofilm. Furthermore, proteins and extracellular DNA have also been found in the matrix.

The nature of the structure of biofilm and the physiologic characteristics of the organisms that inhabit it confer resistance to antimicrobial agents such as antibiotics, disinfectants and detergents. This antimicrobial resistance is not genotypic (i.e. due to plasmids or transposons, or linked to mutational events), but rather due to multicellular strategies and/or the ability of individual cells, in biofilm, to differentiate into a phenotypic state that is resistant to the action of the antibiotic. This resistance is expressed through different mechanisms, such as delayed penetration of the antimicrobial agent through the biofilm matrix; abnormal growth of organisms within the biofilm or physiological changes due to the manner of the biofilm's development. All this explains why only 10% of all microrganisms are distributed, in nature, in planktonic form, a condition that confers "vulnerability" both to attack by phagocytes (macrophages and neutrophils) and to the bacteriostatic and/or bactericidal action of antibiotics.

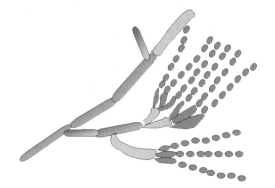

Figure 4.16 Schematic diagram of *Penicillium*.

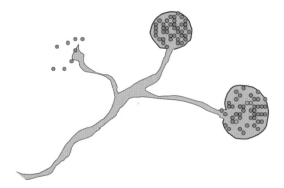

Figure 4.17 Schematic diagram of Zygomycete.

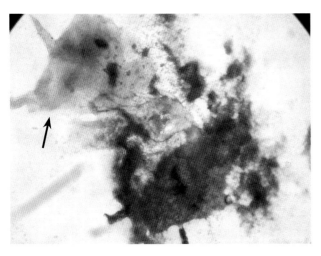

Figure 4.18 Particular "cyan" color in a nasal cytology sample ("infectious spot"; arrow) (MGG staining; ×800).

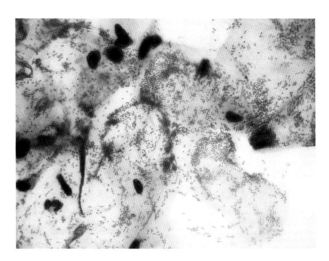

Figure 4.19 "Infectious spot". Initial formation (MGG staining; ×1000).

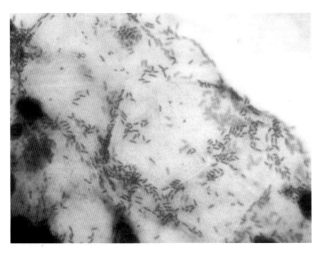

Figure 4.20 "Infectious spot". Particular "cyan" color. Inside, numerous bacteria are visible (MGG staining; ×1000 with CMF 2×).

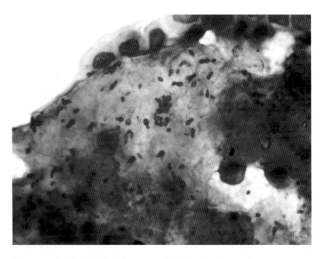

Figure 4.21 "Infectious spot". Bacteria and spores are visible (MGG staining; ×1000 with CMF 2×).

Our recent nasal cytology studies have described, for the first time, certain "morphologic-chromatic" features in patients affected by infectious rhinopathies (bacterial and fungal), and we regard these features as the morphologic-chromatic expression of biofilm.

Crucial to this "chromatism = biofilm" correlation was the finding, in some cytologies, of particular colors, shades of "cyan" (wavelength around 480 nm) that do not usually fall within the color spectrum of a nasal cytology, when the MGG (May-Grumwald-Giemsa) staining method is used (**Fig. 4.18**).

Our suspicion that these chromatic features represented biofilm was strengthened by the fact that we found, almost without exception, within these color formations, the presence of numerous bacteria and/or fungal spores, thus justifying the name "infectious spot" (IS) (**Figs. 4.19-4.23**).

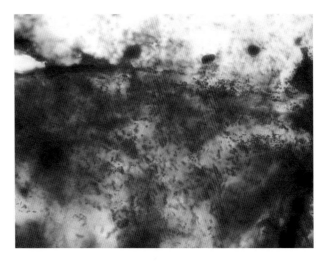

Figure 4.22 "Infectious spot". The stronger color indicates a greater quantity of EPS, and therefore an older biofilm (MGG staining; ×1000 with CMF 2×).

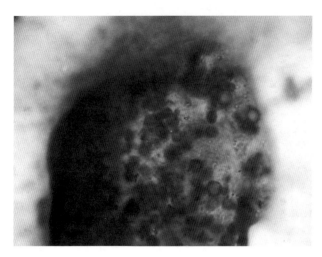

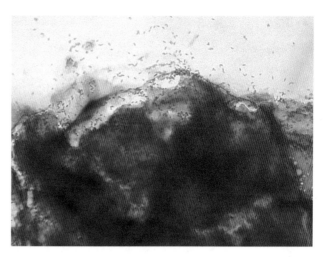

Figure 4.23 "Infectious spot". Typical "tower" appearance of mature biofilm. Bacteria and spores are visible (MGG staining; ×1000 with CMF 4×).

Figure 4.24 "Infectious spot". PAS staining confirms the exopolysaccharidic nature of the infectious spot (MGG staining; ×1000 with CMF 2×).

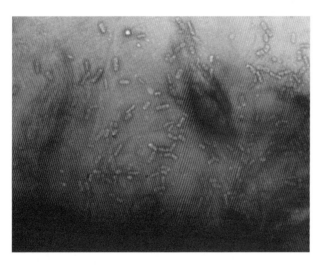

Figure 4.25 "Infectious spot". Same slide as in figure 4.24 at higher magnification. Bacteria are clearly visible embedded in the exopolysaccharide matrix (MGG staining; ×1000 with CMF 4×).

Positive staining with Schiff's reagent (periodic acid staining - Schiff's reagent, PAS), specific for polysaccharides, confirmed the polysaccharidic nature of the matrix of the IS, and, therefore, the fact that it was part of the biofilm (**Figs. 4.24-4.25**).

It should be specified that the IS, while remaining in the spectrum of "cyan", may present varying shades of color, probably due to the age of the biofilm: the older it is, the greater its polysaccharide content and, as a results, the stronger its color (**Figs. 4.19-4.23**).

We believe that these microscopic findings may be helpful, both on a diagnostic level, to further understanding of the microbiologic aspects related to specific rhinopathies (rhinosinusitis, adenoid hypertrophy, nasal polyps, etc.), and on a therapeutic level, for the identification of new drugs and/or medical devices capable of disrupting and/or neutralizing these microbial organizations.

VIRUSES

Viruses are small pathogenic microorganisms, so much smaller than bacteria that they can be seen only by using electron microscopy (**Fig. 4.26**).

Although cytological study using a light microscope does not permit direct observation of the viral agent, light microscopy remains a fundamental diagnostic technique in rhinology because it permits the visualization of the cytopathologic and, in some cases, the pathognomonic effects characteristic of viruses.

The principal viral agents responsible for respiratory conditions are:
- *Myxovirus* influenza groups A, B and C;
- *Paramyxovirus* parainfluenza types 1, 2, 3, 4;
- Respiratory syncytial virus (RSV), comprising 30 serotypes;
- Human *adenovirus*;
- Human *rhinovirus* (of which about 100 serologic types are known);
- *Coronavirus*;
- ECHO (*Enteric cytopathic human orphan*) *virus*.

The herpes viruses (herpes zoster and varicella-zoster virus), A and B Coxsackie viruses and reoviruses are not strictly respiratory viruses, but they may give rise to clinical pictures similar to those induced by the viruses responsible for respiratory infections.

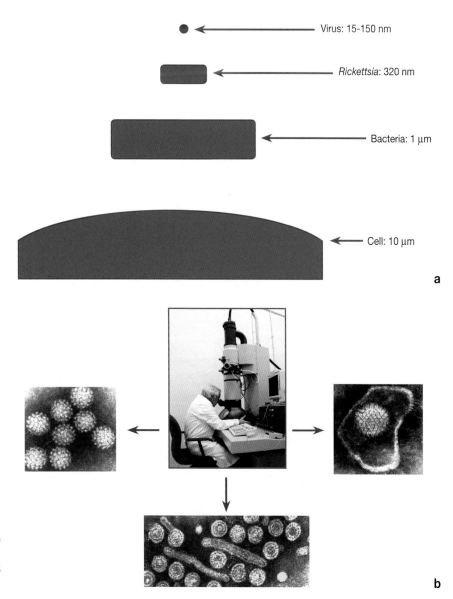

Figure 4.26 Comparison in size of viruses, bacteria and cells (**a**); morphological aspects of viruses (electron microscopy) (**b**).

The Light Microscope

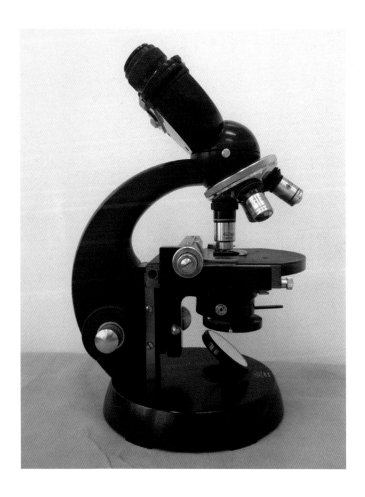

The simplest way to identify cells is by observing them.

J. Tobin

I wish to thank
Nikon Instruments S.p.A. - Italia for their technical assistance
in writing this chapter.

THE STRUCTURE OF THE LIGHT MICROSCOPE

The examination of cells using microscopes dates back to the 17th century but it was not until the late 19th century that cell morphology and function were first described.

Only with the advent of new microscope technologies in the mid-20th century did it become possible to better define the cytoplasm, nucleus and membrane structure of cells (**Fig. 5.1**).

A better appreciation of the numerous scientific applications of microscopy starts with an understanding of the basics of optical physics.

To study the details of an object, we need at least one lens or lens system. If we use a single ten power lens, it will allow us to see the object magnified only ten times (**Fig. 5.2 a**). To overcome this limit, we need a second lens or lens system that can further magnify the image of the magnified object. In brief, this is the principle of microscopy (**Fig. 5.2 b**) which Galileo Galilei tested over 300 years ago. This principle remains as valid today as it was then, and is still the foundation of mechanical and optical developments in microscope technology.

A microscope has the following components (**Fig. 5.3**):
- stand
- ocular lens
- objective lens
- stage
- substage condenser
- field diaphragm
- illuminator.

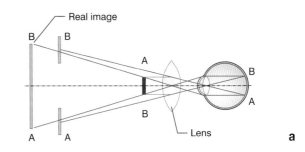

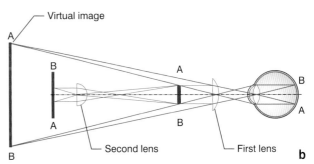

Figure 5.2 Simple optical lens system (**a**); optical principle of a compound microscope (**b**).

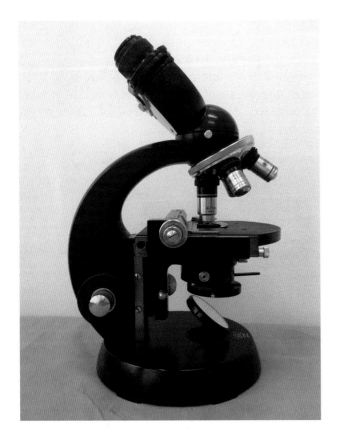

Figure 5.1 Light microscope.

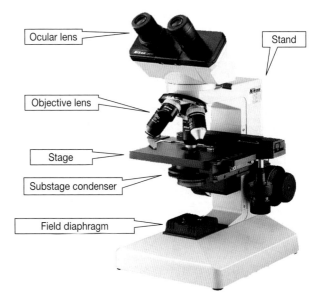

Figure 5.3 Light microscope: structural elements.

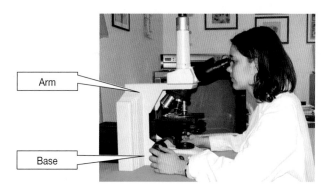

Figure 5.4 Microscope stand.

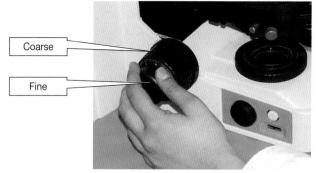

Figure 5.5 Coarse and fine adjustment knobs.

The Microscope Stand

The microscope stand consists of an arm and a base (**Fig. 5.4**). It keeps the instrument stable and holds the control mechanisms for focus adjustment.

Attached to the stand are the coarse and fine adjustment knobs (**Fig. 5.5**) that bring the object into focus and sharpen the focus, respectively.

New models have ergonomically designed stands that incorporate features that permit multiple operations, e.g. moving the cross-travel stage while, at the same time, bringing the object into focus (**Figs. 5.6-5.7**).

The Eyepiece

The eyepiece is a simple lens system that "sees" and magnifies the image of an object already magnified by the objective lens. Older models had monocular, whereas modern ones generally allow more

comfortable binocular viewing that provides better definition.

All eyepieces, comprising two ocular lenses, bear a number etched on the barrel indicating the *magnifying power of the lens* (**Fig. 5.8**). Magnification is calculated by multiplying the magnifying power of the ocular lens by that of the objective lens.

The eye is brought closer to the eyepiece until the point is reached at which the field of vision is largest, i.e. when the light rays from the microscope converge at the point called the *exit pupil* (**Fig. 5.9 a-b**). For operators who wear glasses, there exist special eyepieces where the exit pupil is reached at a greater-than-normal distance. To avoid scratching the lens, eyepieces can be fitted with a rubber collar.

Before a binocular microscope can be used, the *interpupillary distance* between the ocular lenses needs to be adjusted until the right and left visual fields merge (**Fig. 5.10 a-b**).

Even when photomicrographs do not need to be taken, the *diopter* of each ocular lens will still need to be adjusted. This allows the field of vision of the

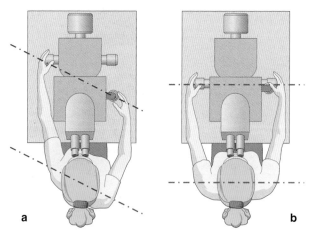

a   b

Figure 5.6 Differences in operator position during coarse and fine adjustment and moving the cross-travel stage. Old generation microscopes (**a**); new generation microscopes (**b**).

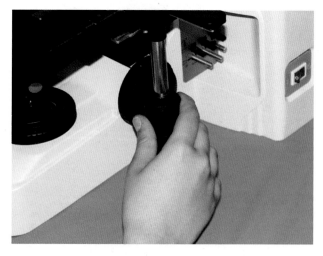

Figure 5.7 Modern microscopes have an ergonomic design that allows the operator to move the cross-travel stage and focus with the same hand.

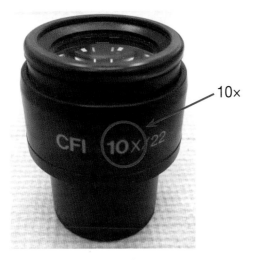

Figure 5.8   Ocular lens (10×).

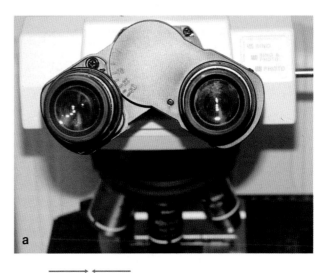

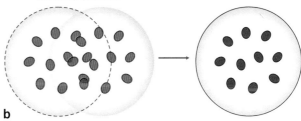

Figure 5.10   Binocular microscope (**a**); adjustment of interpupil distance (**b**).

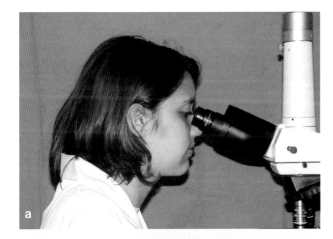

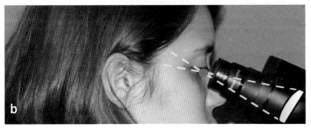

Figure 5.9 a, b   Exit pupil.

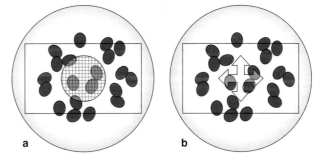

Figure 5.11   Diopter adjustment. Reticle system (**a**); cross system (**b**).

lenses to be focused regardless of differences between the eyes:

- if one of the ocular lenses has a photographic reticle, the adjustment ring must be turned in order to bring the reticle into focus; while doing this, the eye just used must be closed while making the same adjustment using the ring on the other lens; continue, without touching the fine or coarse adjustment knobs, until the specimen is in focus (**Fig. 5.11**);
- if no photographic reticle is mounted on the ocular lens, the specimen is focused first using the right eye (×10-×20 lens); then, with this eye closed and

without touching the coarse or fine adjustment knobs, the adjustment ring on the left ocular lens is rotated until the specimen comes into focus.

The Objective Lens

The objective lens is the most important component of the microscope since the instrument's resolving power, definition and magnifying power are determined by it.

It consists of a system of converging lenses with a short focal distance and projects the magnified in-

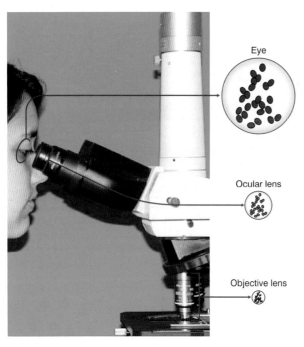

Figure 5.12 Main points of magnification.

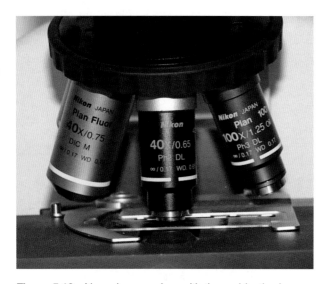

Figure 5.13 Nosepiece revolver with three objective lenses.

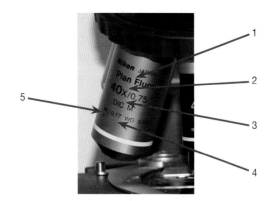

Figure 5.14 Objective lens specifications (see description in the text).

verted image of a specimen onto the lower focal plane of the eyepiece so that it can "see" and further magnify the image (**Fig. 5.12**).

A microscope can have up to six objective lenses with different magnifying powers that are screwed into a revolving nosepiece, or *revolver* (**Fig. 5.13**).

The lens's magnifying power and other important parameters are marked on the barrel.

The objective lens shown in **Figure 5.14**, for example, has the following characteristics:
1) it gives a flat image of the specimen (PLAN);
2) it has a magnifying power of ×40;
3) it can be used for differential interference contrast (DIC) microscopy
4) it requires a coverslip 0.17 mm thick
5) it is infinity corrected (∞).

This last parameter is important because before infinity-corrected objective lenses were introduced, optical tubes came in lengths of either 160 mm or 170 mm, depending on the manufacturer (**Figs. 5.15, 5.16 a**), and the lens system was calculated according to this measurement. This was also why objective lenses could not be used on microscopes produced by different manufacturers. In addition, if the mechanical tube was lengthened with magnification devices, filters, prisms or other intermediate mechanisms, the objective lens became less efficient (**Fig. 5.16 b**).

With modern objectives, however, this problem has been overcome with an optical system calculated to produce an intermediate image at infinity so that the rays of the light beam leaving them are parallel (**Fig. 5.16 c**).

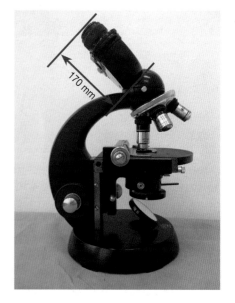

Figure 5.15 Length of optical tube.

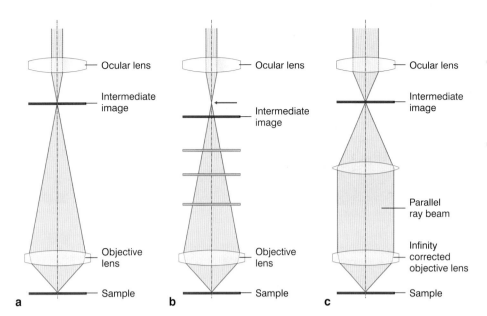

Figure 5.16 Optical tube. Fixed (**a**), variable (**b**), infinity corrected (**c**).

Another important parameter, also marked on the barrel of the objective lens, is the *numerical aperture* (NA) (**Fig. 5.17 a**). This indicates the *resolving power of the objective* and its optical quality.

Numerical aperture is expressed by the formula:

$$NA = n \sin \alpha$$

The beam leaving the specimen and entering the lens is a light cone with an angle width of 2α (**Fig. 5.17 b**). This angle depends on the refractive index (*n*) of the medium between the specimen and the lens.

If the medium is air (*n* = 1), the value of 2α will be low; whereas if cedar oil (*n* = 1.5) is the medium, the value of 2α will be high (**Fig. 5.17 c**).

Thus, the value of 2α indicates the maximum width of the light cone entering the objective lens

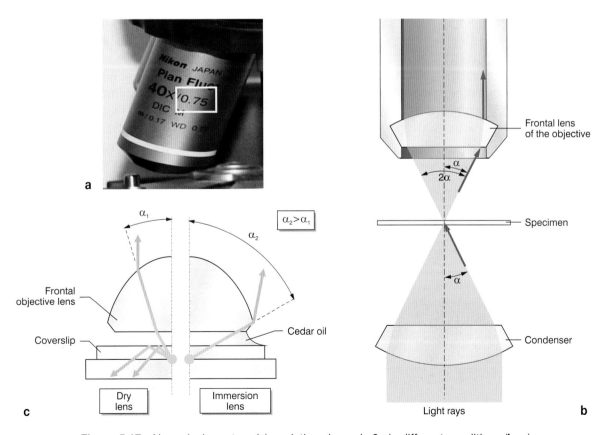

Figure 5.17 Numerical aperture (**a**), variations in angle 2α in different conditions (**b, c**).

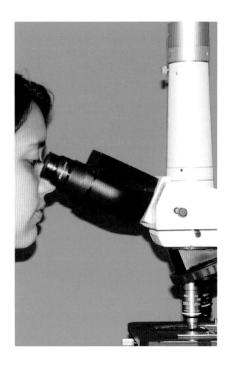

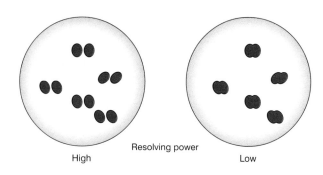

Figure 5.18 Resolving power is the ability to discriminate two particles as separate.

since the NA is directly proportional to the refractive index (n) of the medium between the sample and the objective lens.

Resolving Power

The eye can distinguish two particles as separate only if the two corresponding points in the image formed on the retina fall on two different sensory cells, which must be located at a distance of approximately 5 µm from each other. This is the eye's anatomical limit of resolution, and it corresponds to a distance of about 0.1 mm between the two particles in question: if the two particles are closer together

than this, the eye will confuse them and see them as one. Let us think of an image as consisting of points whose size depends on the physical characteristics of the image itself. The microscope has to be able to enlarge the object until the points that make up its image become visible to the eye, in other words, until a distance of more than 5 µm between one point and the next is reached in the image projected on the retina. Hence, the greater the numerical aperture, the closer the dots can be to one another yet still be seen as separate.

Furthermore, the resolving power (**Fig. 5.18**) is directly proportional to the numerical aperture and the refractive index of the medium between the sample and the objective lens, whereas it is inversely proportional to the wavelength of the light beam. This is why the best objectives are those with a higher numerical aperture, like nearly all immersion lenses.

Placing a liquid (**Fig. 5.19**) between the surface of the specimen and the objective lens produces light rays with a uniform path. With a dry objective lens, the light rays pass through the cover glass ($n = 1.53$), the air ($n = 1.00$) and the lens glass ($n = 1.53$). Whereas with an oil immersion lens, the refractive index of glass can be approached, creating a uniform light path (**Table 5.1**).

Coverslip

Although not a component of the microscope, the coverslip is another factor that influences the

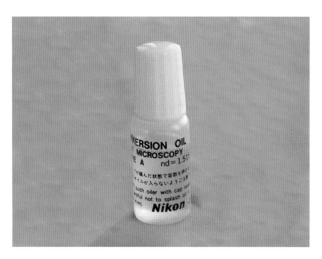

Figure 5.19 Immersion oil.

Table 5.1 Differences in refractive index

Liquid placed between lens and sample	Refractive index (n)
Distilled water	1.33
Glycerin	1.45
Cedar oil	1.51
Synthetic oil	1.51

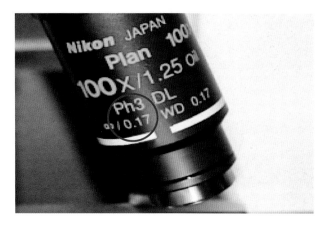

Figure 5.20 Cover glass thickness is always marked on the barrel of the objective lens.

visual quality when viewing a microscopic specimen.

Most histologic and cytologic specimens are mounted on *glass slides* using water, glycerin or synthetic balsam and then covered with an *ultra-thin coverslip*.

The coverslip behaves like a lens with an infinite radius of curvature, i.e. a plane; consequently the coverslip thickness needs to be taken into account when calculating the objective lens power.

Objective lenses are calibrated to accommodate a coverslip thickness of 0.17 mm, so this is marked on the barrel of the objective (**Fig. 5.20**). Unlike immersion lenses, dry lenses are more sensitive to coverslip thickness since they have a higher NA.

Stage

The sample is placed on a stage equipped with slide holders or a cross-travel mechanism (**Fig. 5.21**). The stage is usually rectangular, but it can also be round, fixed or rotatable for polarized light studies or simply to better orientate the specimen.

Since the optical tube is fixed to the microscope stand, the stage and condenser are raised or lowered relative to the objective lens in order to focus on the specimen.

Substage Condenser

All modern microscopes have a substage condenser (**Fig. 5.22**), a lens system that delivers the appropriate amount of light to the objective lens.

The condenser concentrates the light cone coming from the illuminator onto the plane of the specimen. From there it sends the beam to the rear focal plane of the objective. The condenser height must be adjusted and centered to accomplish this.

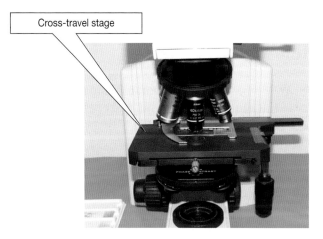

Cross-travel stage

Figure 5.21 Cross-travel stage.

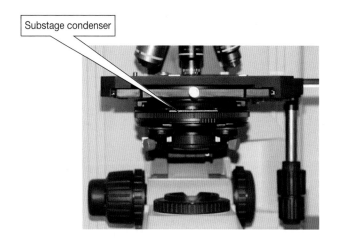

Substage condenser

Figure 5.22 Substage condenser.

The condenser has a shutter diaphragm (aperture diaphragm) that adjusts the light beam to the required NA. By opening or closing the aperture diaphragm as appropriate, the condenser and the objective apertures are optimized.

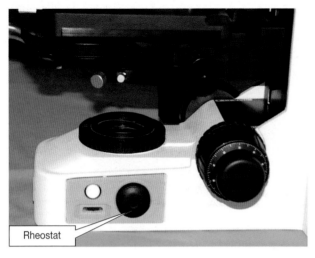

Figure 5.23   Illuminator.

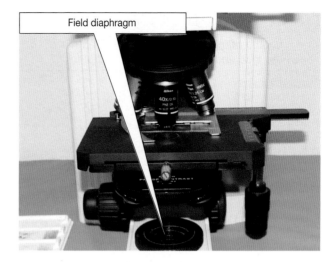

Figure 5.24   Field diaphragm.

Illuminator

An illuminator is incorporated into the design of even the simplest modern microscopes. A low voltage filament lamp is regulated with a rheostat (**Fig. 5.23**).

Field diaphragm

The *field diaphragm*, or illuminator diaphragm, regulates the amplitude of the light beam reaching the condenser and delimits the visual field, thus enhancing image quality (**Fig. 5.24**).

IMAGE ACQUISITION AND ARCHIVING

A comfortable workstation and sufficient counter space are indispensable for looking through a microscope (**Fig. 5.25**).

Having modern equipment at one's disposal is an obvious advantage since recent technological advances have radically changed the methods for acquiring and storing photographic images.

With the advent of digital cameras and dedicated software applications, image acquisition time has been shortened and the quality of high-resolution images has considerably improved.

Scientific digital cameras can be used to take digital photographs and short videos, which are a useful aid in patient follow up and for teaching purposes.

In cytology, digital image systems are also useful because they permit the acquisition of scientific images obtained using microscopic methods *in vivo*,

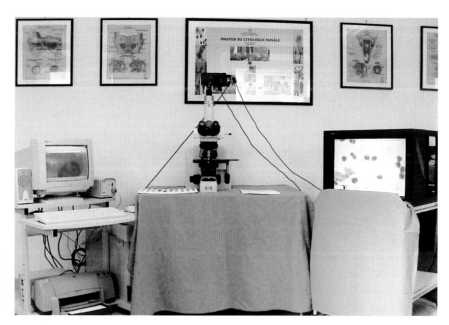

Figure 5.25 Microscope workstation. A digital camera mounted onto a microscope is connected to a computer for acquiring and storing images.

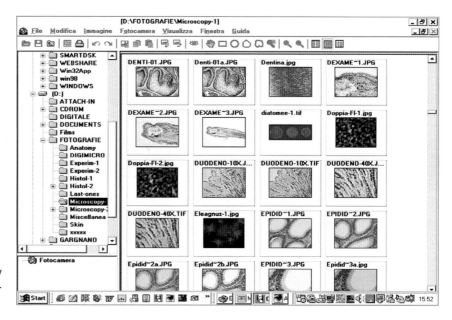

Figure 5.26 Images be can easily managed and stored using dedicated software programs.

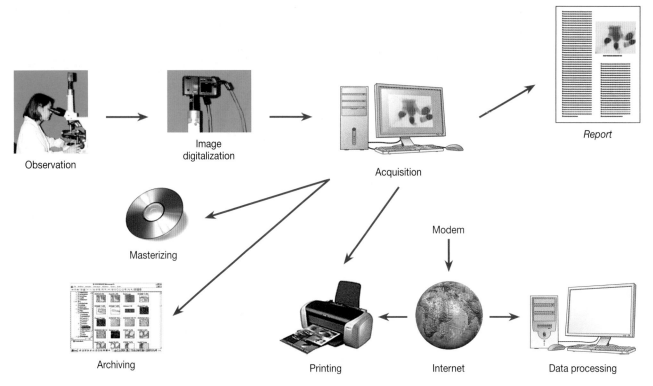

Observation

Image digitalization

Acquisition

Report

Masterizing

Modem

Archiving

Printing

Internet

Data processing

Figure 5.27   Photomicrographs can be archived, printed out, stored on a CD, imported into a report or sent via Internet anywhere around the world for teleconferencing or consultation.

for example, in phase-contrast microscopy or immunofluorescence studies. An additional benefit is that image quality can be checked immediately and the picture retaken if necessary.

Microscopic images can be acquired at basic levels of magnification (×40, ×100, ×400, ×1000), and also further magnified (from ×1.2 to ×4) thanks to the "camera magnification factor" (CMF), an application found on most digital cameras (usually referred to as the "zoom") which allows certain cytologic features to be better highlighted.

Digital photography offers a series of advantages:
- an unlimited number of photographs can be taken;
- there is no cost for acquiring films or developing supplies;
- there are no problems with the choice of film, i.e. black/white or color;

- the images have an unlimited duration as they do not change over time (color, contrast, brightness);
- the images may be reused many times; they are easily stored and retrieved; a CD can hold several hundred images (**Fig. 5.26**);
- real-time image acquisition; immediately after the picture is taken, it can be viewed and retaken if unsuitable;
- it is possible to verify, by direct cross-checking with the specimen, the parameters of perfect photomicroscopy (centered condenser, correct color gradation of light, correct diaphragm closure or aperture at focusing);
- the images can be imported into other software applications (document word processing or presentation softwares, etc.) for presentation at conferences, teleconferences and the classroom (**Fig. 5.27**).

Cytologic Procedures

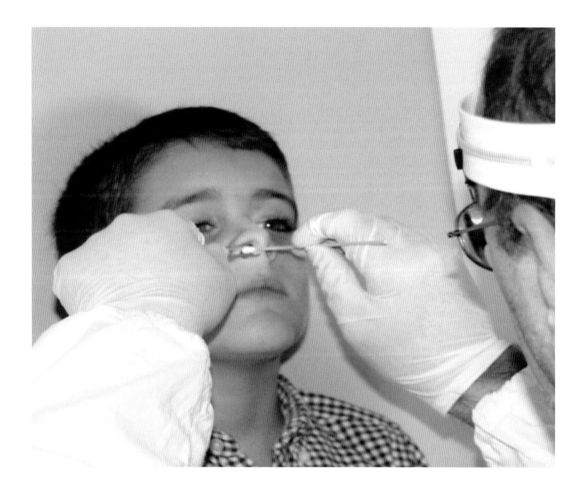

It is true that images are ambiguous. They do not transmit ideas; instead, they stimulate thinking...

Marcel Bessis, 1976

EQUIPMENT AND SUPPLIES

Equipment and supplies for cytologic sampling are inexpensive and readily available (**Fig. 6.1**):
- Head lamp to illuminate the nasal cavity;
- Various sizes of nasal specula (child to adult sizes);
- Sterile nasal cotton tip applicators (throat swabs);
- Rhino-Pro® for nasal scraping;
- Brush for nasal brushing;
- Specimen slides with single frosted end;
- Coverslips;
- Resin for specimen mounting;
- Pencil;
- Adhesive labels;
- Liquid fixatives (see below);
- Staining dyes (see below);
- Slide racks;
- Disposable pipettes;
- Distilled water;
- Disposable gloves;
- Gauze;
- Xylol;

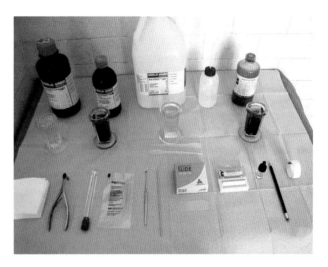

Figure 6.1 Equipment and supplies for cytologic diagnosis.

- Slide box;
- Timer.

How to Take a Cytologic Sample

Before taking a cytologic sample, it is always good practice to explain to the patient what will happen during the procedure. Reassuring the patient helps gain cooperation, particularly in children. Important points to mention are that most procedures, except for biopsy which requires local anesthesia, are quick (a matter of seconds) and painless and do not cause bleeding.

SAMPLING TECHNIQUES

There are many techniques for sampling and processing nasal swabs. Since each has its advantages and disadvantages, the choice of sampling method will depend on what kind of specimen is to be collected. Other factors include patient age, sampling site, thickness of nasal mucosa to be sampled, and the need for repeated sampling for biochemical and bacteriologic studies.

Nose Blowing

For the patient, nose blowing is a simple and painless way to produce a sample. Cytologic study is performed on the nasal secretions collected onto waxed paper or plastic wrap (**Fig. 6.2**) and then spread on a microscopic slide. The limitations to this method include the following:
- the nasal secretion is poorly representative of the cell population; ciliated cells are rarely present;
- the nasal secretion will contain only some of the cells normally present in the nasal epithelium but many exfoliated cells;
- bacterial contamination by the saprophytic bacteria normally residing in the nostrils;

- low quality staining because of excessive mucus that obscures the field of view.

Other problems are that very young children may not know how to blow their nose or that adults with atrophic disorders may not be able to supply enough secretion for the examination.

Nasal Lavage

Like nose blowing, nasal lavage is a non-invasive procedure in which a small amount of saline solution (0.9% NaCl) is introduced into the nasal cavities and the return lavage fluid is collected in a test tube and centrifuged (300 rpm for 10 min). The resulting pellet is then suspended in 1 ml saline solution for performing a cell count with a hemocytometer (**Fig. 6.3**).

Alternatively, the sample is centrifuged at 700 rpm for 5 min (Cytospin) and then left to air dry before staining as required.

Although apparently simpler than other sampling methods, nasal lavage entails several extra steps (centrifuging, supernatant suspension, Cytospin, etc.) that render it less practical in an outpatient setting.

Another disadvantage is that it yields few mucosal

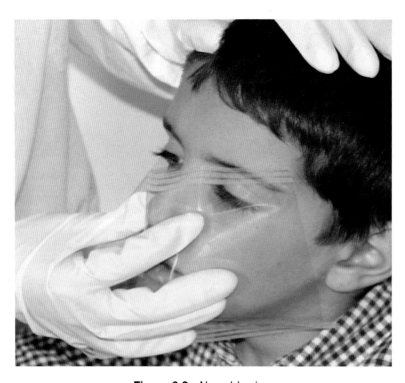

Figure 6.2 Nose blowing.

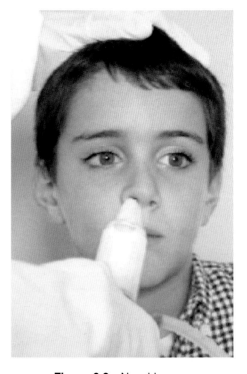

Figure 6.3 Nasal lavage.

epithelial cells (goblet cells, ciliated cells, etc.) and a predominance of squamous cells of the nasal vestibule and cells contained in the mucus (neutrophils, bacteria, eosinophils, etc.) (**Fig. 6.4**).

Nasal Swabbing

Nasal swabbing is a simple way to collect cells from epithelial secretions.

Using a sterile cotton tip applicator (throat swab) moistened with saline solution, the nasal mucosa is swabbed gently to prevent damaging cell material (**Fig. 6.5**).

The sample is taken from the middle portion of the inferior turbinate by delicately rotating the swab back and forth and up and down for about 4 to 5 seconds.

As with nose blowing, sample cell count will vary considerably. Nonetheless, this technique is a useful aid for determining the ratios of specific cell populations.

Moreover, since it is safe and relatively quick to perform, this method is usually recommended in uncooperative children or circumstances where nasal brushing or scraping may be unacceptable to the patient.

Nasal Brushing

Nasal brushing is performed using small brushes with nylon bristles (**Fig. 6.6**). The brush is advanced between the septum and the inferior turbinate and then rotated as it is withdrawn from the nose. This will create transient discomfort for the patient. The collection includes cells from the secretion and the epithelial surface.

The material is precipitated in a sterile solution and centrifuged; the resulting supernatant is then transferred to a glass slide for fixing and staining.

Nasal Scraping

Nasal scraping is the best method for obtaining a representative sample of nasal mucosal cells.

It can be performed as a non-invasive procedure that causes the patient minor discomfort.

The first step is to have the patient blow his nose to eliminate excess secretion. Then, under direct visual inspection, the uppermost layer of the mucosa is sampled using a Rhino-Pro® or similar type of curette (**Fig. 6.7**) while taking care not to cause bleeding.

In this way, the cells collected from the epithelial

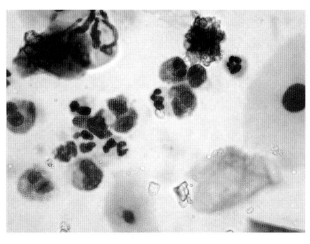

Figure 6.4   Nasal lavage. The specimen shows numerous immuno-inflammatory cells (eosinophils, neutrophils, lymphocytes) and squamous epithelial cells of the nasal vestibule. Ciliated and goblet cells are absent (Allergic rhinitis; MGG staining; ×1000).

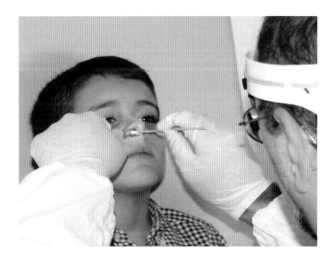

Figure 6.5   Nasal swabbing.

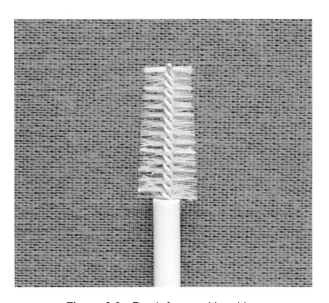

Figure 6.6   Brush for nasal brushing.

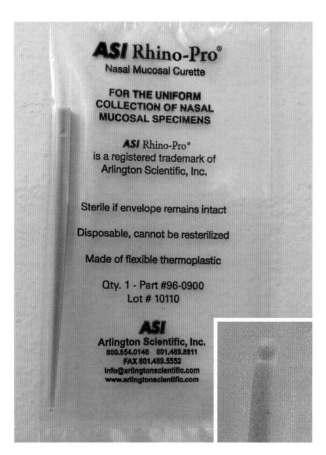

Figure 6.7 Rhino-Pro® and sterile disposable package.

lining are well preserved and can be used for differential diagnosis.

The sample is spread uniformly in the center of the slide, again taking care not to squash or damage the cells.

The advantages to this technique are that it causes the patient only minor discomfort (it doesn't require anesthesia) and can be repeated as needed.

In addition, the sample can be further used for bacteriology or virology studies and biochemical or immunohistochemical determinations.

Finally, our recent studies have shown that this sampling method is also suitable for studying the ultrastructure of the ciliary apparatus.

Biopsy

Strictly speaking, biopsy is a histologic rather than a cytologic technique. Biopsy permits complete examination of the mucosa and the tunica propria. The drawbacks are that it is painful, and thus requires anesthesia, and that it may cause serious bleeding, sometimes so severe as to require the use of a nasal swab to achieve temporary hemostasis.

SAMPLING SITES

As mentioned above, common sampling sites are the inferior (middle third portion) and the middle turbinates since they provide diagnostically reliable samples (**Fig. 6.8**).

The superior turbinate is rarely sampled because it is difficult to visualize and because of the risk of nasovagal reflex. Sampling of the nasal septal mucosa is inadvisable because it yields poorly representative samples and because of the high risk of a profuse nosebleed due to the rich vasculature.

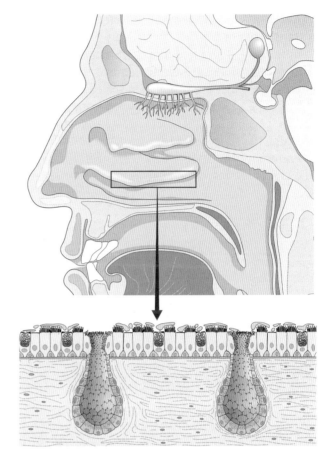

Figure 6.8 Main sampling site: middle third portion of the inferior turbinate.

SWAB PROCESSING

After the sample has been collected, the material is transferred to a microscope slide.

In the past, slides had to be scrupulously cleaned with special slide cleaners to remove dust. Today, microscope slides are supplied in sealed boxes ready for use. The slide should be removed from the package as needed and handled by its edge to avoid touching the slide surface.

Preferably the slide will have a frosted area at one end (**Fig. 6.9**) where the patient's name, sampling date and other data can be written. This should be done using a pencil so as to avoid causing alterations during fixation, staining, washing, etc.

The sample should be visible to the naked eye (**Fig. 6.10**) but not too thick. A fine monolayer can be achieved by spreading the mucus on the slide with a thin disposable loop.

After the cytologic smear has been prepared, it is ready for fixation.

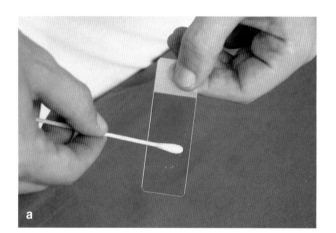
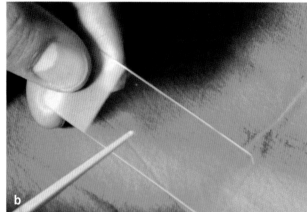

Figure 6.9 Nasal smear. Nasal swab (**a**); Rhino-Pro® (**b**).

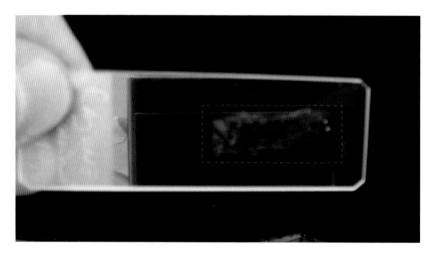

Figure 6.10 The smear should be clearly visible to the naked eye yet not too thick.

FIXATION

Air drying is not a fixation method per se since no liquid fixer is used, however, air-dried specimens may still be considered fixed as cells do not undergo hemolysis in the absence of water. Specimens can be dried almost instantly by preheating the slide (40 °C) or drying the specimen under an infrared lamp.

There are numerous fixation methods (**Table 6.1**). Air dying is recommended only if the specimen is to be stained within a couple of hours. Other techniques use acetone, unscented hair spray, Mota's basic lead acetate, 95% ethyl alcohol and ether (1:1).

The specimen may also be fixed with absolute methyl alcohol and left to react for 3 min. However, when MGG stain is used, the dye itself acts as a fixative because it is diluted in alcohol.

After fixation, the specimen is ready for staining. If staining is to be done later, the specimen can be stored for up to two days in a closed container to protect it from dust, fungal spores or other airborne particulates.

Table 6.1 Fixation methods

- Air drying
  (recommended for MGG staining)
- Acetone
- Unscented hair spray
- Mota's basic lead acetate
- Buffered formalin
- Methyl alcohol
- 95% ethyl alcohol
- 95% ethyl alcohol in ether (1:1)

STAINING

Staining is a procedure whereby a dye or combination of dyes and reagents is used to color the components of cells. In this way, a cell's degree of maturity, type, state of function and any involutional phenomena can be detected.

In addition, staining permits the study of the enzymatic composition of the cell's components and cytochemical structure in relation to growth stage and function. There is a wide variety of dyes and staining techniques. The choice will depend on specimen requirements (**Table 6.2**).

May-Grünwald-Giemsa (MGG), the most commonly used stain in cytology, demonstrates the cell types frequently found in the nasal mucosa.

May-Grünwald-Giemsa (MGG) Staining

The slide, with the specimen facing up, is placed in a well. Several of drops of May-Grünwald dye are applied to cover the entire surface and allowed to react for 3 min. This will fix the specimen but not yet stain it as dyes in methyl alcohol are not ionized.

Table 6.2 Staining techniques

Dyes	Cell type
Hansel's	Eosinophils
Wright's	Basophils
Wright-Giemsa	Eosinophils, basophils, neutrophils, mast cells
Papanicolaou	Exfoliated epithelial cells, nuclear and cytoplasmic organelles
Toluidine blue	Basophils and mast cells
Leishman's	Eosinophils
Alcian yellow	Mast cells
Randolph's	Eosinophils
Alcian blue	Basophils and mast cells
May-Grünwald	Neutrophils

The slide is then treated with buffered water (the same amount as the dye) for 6 min. The slide is taken from the well, rinsed in distilled water without

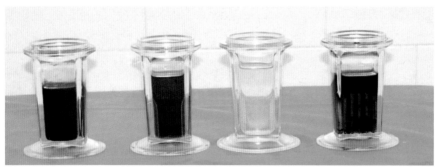

| May-Grünwald pure (3 min) | May-Grünwald diluted 1:1 (6 min) | Distilled water (1 min) | Giemsa diluted 1:10 (30 min) |

Figure 6.11 May-Grünwald-Giemsa (MGG) staining.

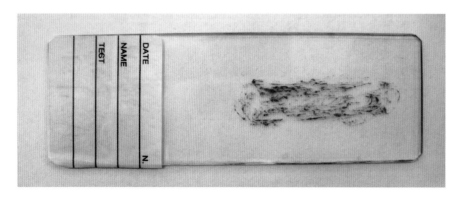

Figure 6.12 Stained slide specimen.

excessively washing it, to remove the stain, and dipped in Giemsa solution. In the meantime, the preparation has stained blue.

The Giemsa solution should be diluted 1:10 with buffered water. The slide is left in the solution for about 20-30 min. Special jars should be used that allow the slides to stand upright. This prevents precipitation that would otherwise result in suboptimal microscopic viewing (**Fig. 6.11**).

After removal from the Giemsa solution, the slide is washed under running water (cells do not usually run away) and left to dry (**Fig. 6.12**).

Figure 6.11 gives the standard reaction times for each solution. However, staining will depend on many factors, including smear thickness, reagent dilution, room temperature, and pH of the distilled water. Some dyes require buffered water. As a general rule, staining should be checked under the microscope every 5-7 min. An indication of successful staining is when the cell nuclei turn pink-violet.

Effects of MGG Staining

- Nuclei stain red violet (*basichromatin*) and pink (*oxychromatin*)
- Basophilic cytoplasm stains from sky blue to dark blue
- Acidophilic cytoplasm stains pink
- Neutrophilic granules stain tan and pink (mixture of granulation)
- Acidophilic granules stain orange
- Basophilic granules (metachromatic) stain dark violet
- Azurophilic granules stain purple or violet-purple
- Erythrocyte basophilic granules stain cobalt blue (**Fig. 6.13 a-b**).

Staining with this technique does not demonstrate mitochondria or centrioles. Since the centrosome is colorless, it can be located in the presence of intense cytoplasmic staining.

It should be kept in mind that stains may be altered because of dye age or poor quality or water that is too acidic or too alkaline. To verify whether the resulting colors are correct, they should be compared with the standard staining colors of known cell components.

For example, an overly blue smear may result from insufficient washing, prolonged staining, high alkalinity of the dye, the water, or the buffer, or a smear that is too thick. In this case, lymphocytic cytoplasm stains gray or lavender, neutrophilic granules appear voluminous and dark, and eosinophilic granules look gray or brown.

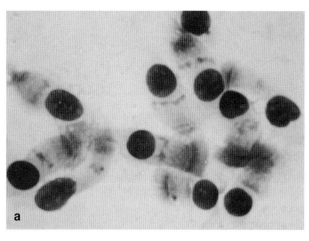

a

Cell component		Staining
Cytoplasm		Basophilic: from sky blue to dark blue; Acidophilic: pink
Nucleus		Red-violet (basochromatin) and pink (oxychromatin)
Mucosal secretion		Basophilic: from sky blue to dark blue; Acidophilic: pink-violet
Neutrophilic granules (Neutrophils)		Beige-pale pink
Acidophilic granules (Eosinophils)		Orange
Basophilic granules (Mast cells)		Dark violet
Bacteria		Dark blue
Fungal spores		Violet with peripheral enhancement

b

Figure 6.13 Numerous ciliated cells with evident supra-nuclear hyperchromatic stria (SHS+) (MGG staining; ×1000 with CMF 1.2×) (**a**); cell components and staining characteristics. MGG dye (**b**).

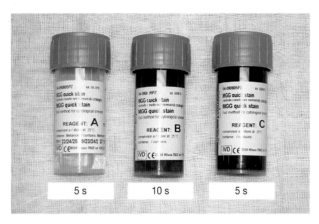

Figure 6.14 MGG Quick Stain®: quick staining kit (Bio Optica Milan, Italy).

An overly red smear may mean that the dye, the buffer, or the water was too acidic. The nuclear chromatin appears red instead of violet, and the eosinophilic granules stain bright red.

Given these possible pitfalls, it is always a good idea to use a timer to signal the staining times, so as to avoid the risk of inadvertently leaving cytologic slides in dyes, which is easily done when one is taken up by other duties, medical or otherwise (for example administrative-bureaucratic tasks).

Less commonly used dyes are *toluidine blue* and *hematoxylin and eosin stain*.

For a few years now, rapid staining kits have been available on the market (MGG Quick Stain®; **Fig. 6.14**). The dyes present in the solutions supplied with these kits are the same ones used in the formulation of traditional MGG solutions. The rapidity with which the staining process is accomplished using these kits (20 seconds) is due to the degree of dissociation of the active chemical species (eosin and thiazine dyes), which speeds up their absorption by the cell structures.

It is important to immerse and remove the slide as specified in the method. Leaving the slide in the staining solution will not guarantee good staining.

Toluidine Blue

Toluidine blue is a metachromatic dye. On contact with chromotropic substances (e.g. acid muco-polysaccharides in basophilic granulocytes), it turns from its orthochromatic color (pale blue) to reddish-purple (**Fig. 6.15 a-c**).

REAGENTS
- 30% ethanol in distilled water;
- 95% ethanol; 0.1% solution in 30% methanol;
- Toluidine blue.

PROCEDURE
- Air dry the smear;
- Dip the slide in toluidine blue solution for 5 min;
- Wash in 95% ethanol and air dry;
- Observe the slide at high-power magnification using an immersion lens.

The nuclei should all stain pale blue, while the mucopolysaccharides should appear wine-red demonstrating basophilic leukocytic granules (metachromatic reaction).

Hematoxylin and Eosin Stain (H&E)

Hematoxylin is an selective dye of the nuclear chromatin. It provides good contrast with the reddish-orange cytoplasmic staining obtained using eosin (**Fig. 6.16**). H&E is normally used in histologic preparations, while the Papanicolaou method is preferred for cytologic studies. The two methods work according to the same principle.

REAGENTS
- Commercially available hematoxylin;
- Commercially available eosin;
- Acidulated water or acidulated alcohol (HCl 2‰ in water or 70% alcohol);
- Lithium carbonate (2‰ solution saturated in H_2O or in 70% alcohol).

PROCEDURE
- Hydrate the fixed preparations in distilled water;
- Stain with hematoxylin for 1-3 min and check results under the microscope;
- Rinse under running water for 1 min;
- Remove excess stain by dipping the slide in water or acidulated alcohol until the dye no longer streaks;

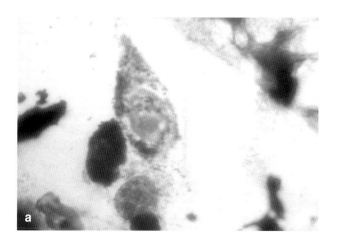
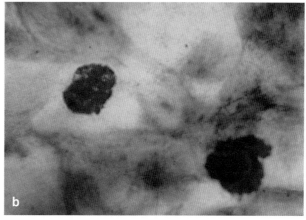
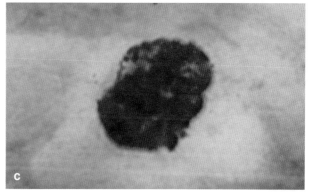

Figure 6.15 a-c Toluidine blue staining demonstrates metachromasia in mast cell granules.

- Rinse under running water;
- Treat with lithium carbonate for 1 min;
- Rinse in distilled water (10-15 immersions);
- Stain with eosin (4-5 immersions);
- Rinse under tap water for at least 1 min;
- Dehydrate with alcohol, clear with xylol or toluol and then mount using balsam or resin.

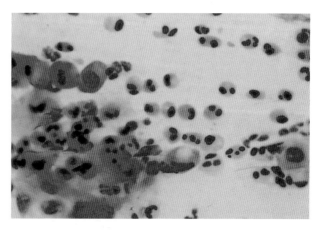

Figure 6.16 Hematoxylin and eosin (H&E) stain (×1000).

SLIDE MOUNTING

The slide needs to be mounted before the specimen can be viewed under the microscope.

The procedure entails (**Fig. 6.17**):

- applying a resin to secure the coverslip to the slide;
- applying an adhesive label indicating the patient's name and the date of sample collection.

During microscopic viewing, all relevant observations should be noted on a data collection form. Once the examination is complete, the slide should be cleaned and placed in a slide holder (**Figs. 6.18-6.20**).

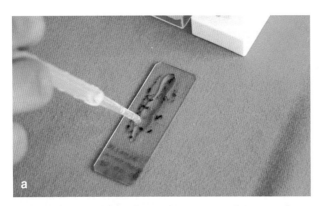

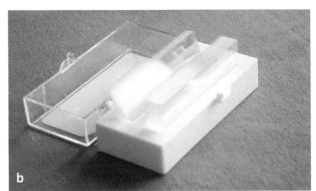

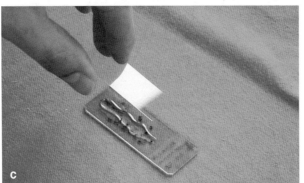

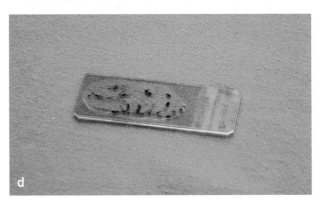

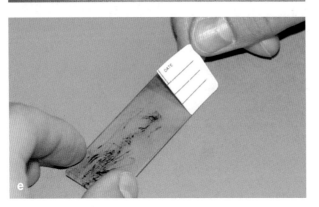

Figure 6.17 Slide mounting. Applying resin (**a**); slide box (**b**); applying coverslip (**c-d**); applying adhesive label with date and patient's data (**e**).

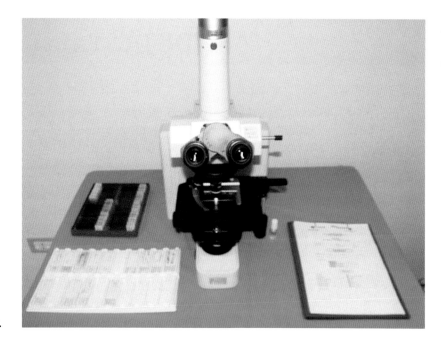

Figure 6.18 Microscope workstation.

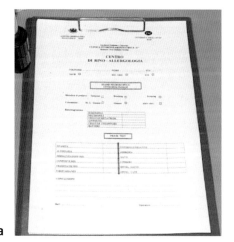

a

Figure 6.19 Data collection form (a); grid for cell counting (for use see Figure 6.26) (b).

Nasal cytology: grid for semiquantitative analysis						
	Microscopic field (immersion, ×1000)	o........ I........10 ....I........20........I........30........I........40........I........50				
	0 NO	+ (occasional)	++ (moderate)	+++ (many)	++++ (large number)	
Ciliated cells	0	20 20 20 20 20	20 20 20 20 20	20 20 20 20 20	20 20 20 20 20	SHS + % CCP % PNL %
Caliciform mucous cells	0	20 20 20 20 20	20 20 20 20 20	20 20 20 20 20	20 20 20 20 20	
Metaplasia	0	20 20 20 20 20	20 20 20 20 20	20 20 20 20 20	20 20 20 20	
Neutrophils	0	11 11 11 11 11 / 11 11 11 11 11	11 11 11 11 11 / 11 11 11 11 11	20 20 20	20 20 20	
Eosinophils	0	1 1 1 1 1	1 1 1 1 1	11 11 11 11 11 / 11 11 11 11 11	11 11 11 11 11 / 11 11 11 11 11	Degr. 0
Mast cells	0	1 1 1 1 1	1 1 1 1 1	11 11 11 11 11 / 11 11 11 11 11	11 11 11 11 11 / 11 11 11 11 11	Degr. 0
Lymphocytes	0	1 1 1 1 1	1 1 1 1 1	11 11 11 11 11 / 11 11 11 11 11	11 11 11 11 11 / 11 11 11 11 11	Act. %
Bacteria	0	I I I	II II	III III / III	IIIIIIIIIIIIIIIIIIIII / IIIIIIIIIIIIIIIIIIIII	Intra 0 Extra 0
Spores	0	I I I	II II	III III / III	IIIIIIIIIIIIIIIIIIIII / IIIIIIIIIIIIIIIIIIIII	Hyphae 0 IS 0

b

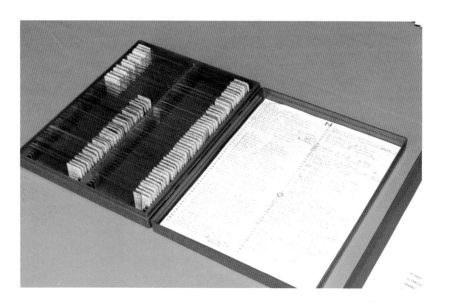

Figure 6.20 Slide holder.

SLIDE DESTAINING

Slides need to be destained before they can be reused for further examinations to demonstrate additional specimen features.

The coverslip can be detached from the slide with xylol. This is done by cooling the slide (–10° C to –20° C) in an upright position for several minutes to several hours. The coverslip should not be forced off as this may damage the preparation.

After removing the coverslip, the slide is rinsed by repeated immersion in xylol and then gradually rehydrated in decreasing concentrations of alcohol and then distilled water.

The slide is then dipped in hydrochloric alcohol (100 ml 70% ethyl alcohol + 1 ml concentrated hydrochloric acid) for 2 to 60 min. The degree of destaining is checked under the microscope. The slide is then rinsed in distilled water.

A slide can seldom be completely destained and some cell damage is inevitable. However, when done carefully, this procedure permits reuse of the slide for many other purposes, particularly for immunofluorescence and immunohistochemical studies.

PITFALLS AND TROUBLESHOOTING

Many potential pitfalls can be encountered in the course of sampling and swab processing (**Fig. 6.21**).

An inadequate preparation may occur as the result of a smear that is too thick. Also if a smear is handled roughly the cells can undergo cytolysis leading to artifacts that make interpretation of the specimen difficult.

Too much mucus may obscure the epithelial cells, just as too many neutrophils will obscure other important details.

Another factor is the ambient air quality of the workplace. An open window is a likely source of contamination with pollen or other airborne particles (**Fig. 6.22**).

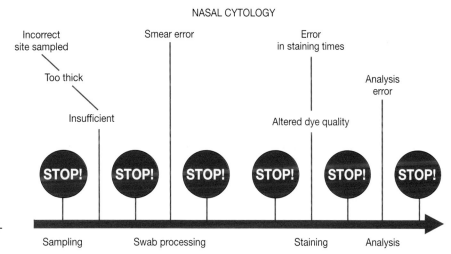

Figure 6.21 Common pitfalls leading to inadequate smears.

Table 6.3 **Troubleshooting of common problems**

Problem	Solution
Smear too thick	Spread material in a thin layer
Smear-related artifacts	Spread material delicately
Too much mucus	Have the patient clean or blow his nose before taking the sample. Remember: cytologic study is performed on the nasal mucosa and not on the mucus
Inadequate fixation	Fix the preparation if it is not to be stained the same day
Presence of erythrocytes	Take the sample under close visual control and without excessive force. Tell the patient what will be done prior to the next step of the procedure The patient's head should be held perfectly still during sampling
Inadequate staining	Keep track of staining times for the specific method used Use a timer with an alarm
Smear contaminated with:	
• airborne dust, spores and pollen	Store stained slides in closable containers
• iron debris	Always use distilled water to stain slides
• bacteria	Avoid touching the skin of the nasal vestibule during sampling since it is usually colonized by saprophytic bacteria, particularly in children

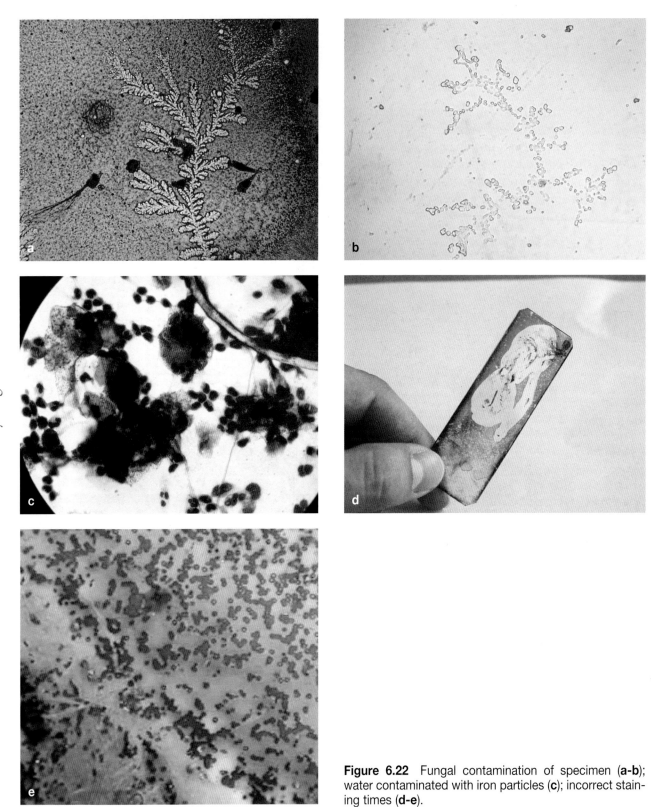

Figure 6.22 Fungal contamination of specimen (**a-b**); water contaminated with iron particles (**c**); incorrect staining times (**d-e**).

The easiest way to avoid these and similar problems is to take the necessary precautions and to pay close attention to timing each step correctly (**Table 6.3**).

MICROSCOPIC OBSERVATION

Cytologic analysis should be performed by qualified or trained personnel. Operators should be able to appreciate the finest differences between normal and abnormal findings. In recognizing abnormal findings they should also be able to identify the elements for a differential diagnosis.

A major difficulty in interpreting nasal cytograms is that no standardized analytic method exists for doing cell counts.

One method is to count the number of cells per field, first viewing the entire slide to find the cell types usually most useful for diagnosis (eosinophils,

mast cells, neutrophils, bacteria, spores, infectious spots, etc.).

The next step is to gain a general impression of the specimen by scanning the slide with a low-power lens (×10), evaluating staining quality and cell distribution (**Fig. 6.23 a**).

Then, having identified an area of greater cell concentration or distribution, the specimen can be viewed using a lens with higher magnifying power (×40) (**Fig. 6.23 b**). But the real analytic assessment begins with high-power magnification (×1000) with an oil immersion lens (**Fig. 6.23 c**).

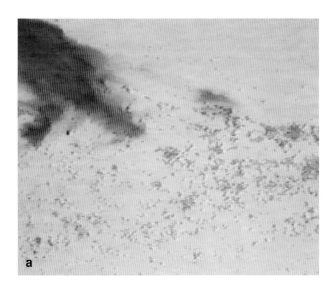

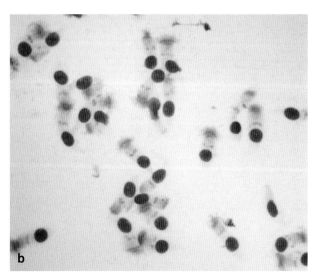

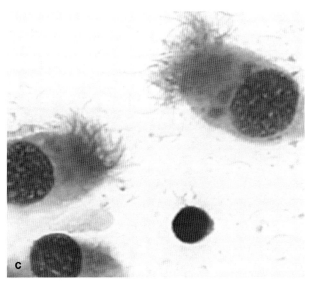

Figure 6.23 View at ×100 (**a**); view at ×400 (**b**); view at ×1000 (oil immersion) (**c**) (MGG staining; CMF 2×).

Table 6.4   Nasal cytogram analysis

	Quantitative analysis	Semiquantitative analysis	Grade
Epithelial cells	N/A	Normal morphology	N
	N/A	Abnormal morphology	A
	N/A	Ciliocytophthoria and/or multinucleation	CCP/MNC
Caliciform mucous (goblet) cells**	0	None	0
	1-24%	Occasional to few cells	1 +
	25-49%	Moderate number	2 +
	50-74%	Many cells easily seen	3 +
	75-100%	Large number, may cover the entire field	4 +
Neutrophils and eosinophils	0	None	0
	0.1-1.0*	Occasional cells	1/2 +
	1.1-5.0*	Few scattered cells or small clumps	1 +
	5.1-15.0*	Moderate number of cells and larger clumps	2 +
	15.1-20.0*	Larger clumps of cells that do not cover the entire field	3 +
	> 20*	Larger clumps of cells covering the entire field	4 +
Basophilic cells	0*	None	0
	0.1-0.3*	Occasional cells	1/2 +
	0.4-1.0*	Few scattered cells	1 +
	1.1-3.0*	Moderate number of cells	2 +
	3.1-6.0*	Many cells easily seen	3 +
	>6.0*	Large number of cells, up to 25 per high-power field	4 +
Eosinophil/mast cell degranulation	Present/absent	Not seen	0
		Occasional granules	1+
		Moderate number of granules	2+
		Many granules easily seen	3+
		Massive degranulation covering the entire field	4+
Bacteria	N/A	None seen	0
	N/A	Occasional clumps	1 +
	N/A	Moderate number	2 +
	N/A	Many easily seen	3 +
	N/A	Large numbers covering the entire field	4 +
Fungal spores	N/A	None seen	0
	N/A	Occasional clumps	1 +
	N/A	Moderate number	2 +
	N/A	Many spores easily seen	3 +
	N/A	Large numbers of spores covering the entire field	4 +
Infectious spot	Present/absent	Present/absent	Present/absent

N denotes normal, A abnormal, CCP ciliocytophthoria, MNC multinucleation; * mean of cells per 10 high-power fields (×1000); ** ratio of goblet to epithelial cells.
Original data from Meltzer EO, et al, 1999 (adapted).

Quantitative Analysis

Having established the site of observation and cell counting, a drop of immersion oil (**Fig. 5.19**) is placed on the area in question and the cells in each field are counted through a high-power lens (×1000).

The mean count of each cell population over ten fields is then calculated. This can be expressed as the proportion of one cell population with respect to another or to the total population.

Semiquantitative Analysis and Grading

It is helpful to complete the cytologic observation reporting the results of semiquantitative analysis and the degree of inflammation based on the values given in appropriate reference tables (**Table 6.4**).

It is also useful to evaluate the presence of bacteria (intra- and extracellular), the bacterial morphology (cocci, rods), cell changes (ciliary apparatus, cytoplasm, nucleus) and the presence of spores or fungal hyphae.

An example of a grading table that correlates cell type with various forms of rhinitis is given in **Table 6.5**.

With a view to arriving at a standardization of nasal cytogram sampling procedures and interpretation, I recently proposed, to the members of the Italian Academy of Nasal Cytology (AICNA), that we adhere to the following specifications:
- the cell sample should be spread over a precise area of the slide (**Fig. 6.24**);
- at least 50 high-power fields (×1000) in immersion should be evaluated (**Fig. 6.25**);
- for cell counting, and the relative semi-quantitative analysis, the criteria shown in figure 6.26 should be adopted.

Table 6.5 Cell types in various nasal diseases

Cell population	Diagnostic classification
Increased eosinophils (1+ to 4+)	Allergic rhinitis
	NARES (Non Allergic Rhinitis with Eosinophilia Syndrome)
	NARESMA (Non Allergic Rhinitis with Eosinophils and Mast Cells) if associated with mast cells
	Aspirin sensitivity
	Nasal polyposis
	Widal's syndrome (nasal polyposis + asthma + aspirin sensitivity)
Increased neutrophils (2+ to 4+)	
• with extra- and intracellular bacteria and infectious spots	Rhinosinusitis/Rhinoadenoiditis
• with ciliocytophthoria and/or multinucleation	Viral rhinitis
• with spores and hyphae and possibly infectious spots	Fungal rhinitis (usually secondary to bacterial infection, associated with nasal polyposis or immunosuppression - AIDS)
• without bacteria	Inflammatory rhinitis (physiochemical stimuli)
	NARNE (Non Allergic Rhinitis with Neutrophils)
	Antrochoanal polyps
Increased basophils (1+ to 4+)	NARMA (Non Allergic Rhinitis with Mast Cells) (nasal mastocytosis)
	Allergic rhinitis (pollen-induced forms)
	Aspirin sensitivity
	Nasal polyposis
	Widal's syndrome (nasal polyposis + asthma + aspirin sensitivity)
Increased eosinophils and basophils in a non allergic patient (1+ to 4+)	NARESMA (Non Allergic Rhinitis with Eosinophils and Mast Cells)

Original data from Meltzer EO, Jalowayski AA, 1988 (adapted).

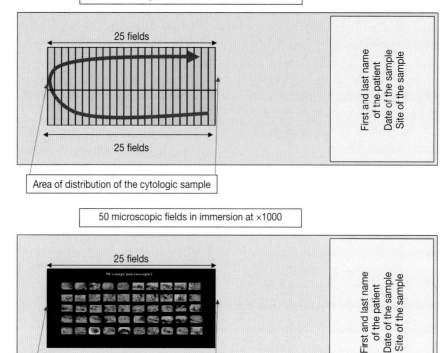

Figure 6.24 Distribution of the cytologic sample on the slide and its subdivision into microscopic fields (**a**); to proceed with cell counting it is necessary to obtain, using a camera attached to the microscope, 50 microscopic images at ×1000, in immersion. This procedure, proposed to AICNA (the Italian Academy of Nasal Cytology), facilitates not only cell counting, but also the storing of the images from each patient (**b**).

Nasal cytology: semiquantitative analysis						
		Microscopic field (immersion, ×1000)	o........ I........10 ....I........20.......I........30.......I........40.......I........50			
	0 NO	+ (occasional)	++ (moderate)	+++ (many)	++++ (large number)	
Ciliated cells	0	1-100	101-200	210-300	>300	SHS + % CCP % PNL %
Caliciform mucous cells	0	1-100	101-200	210-300	>300	
Metaplasia	0	1-100	101-200	210-300	>300	
Neutrophils	0	1-20	21-40	41-100	>100	
Eosinophils	0	1-5	6-10	11-30	>30	Degr. 0
Mast cells	0	1-5	6-10	11-30	>30	Degr. 0
Lymphocytes	0	1-5	6-10	11-30	>30	Act. %
Bacteria	0	I I I	II II	III III III																								
																										Intra 0 Extra 0
Spores	0	I I I	II II	III III III																								
																										Hyphae 0 IS 0

Figure 6.25 Semiquantitative analysis of the nasal cytogram. SHS, supranuclear hyperchromatic striae; CCP, ciliocytophthoria; PNL, polynucleation; Degr., degranulation; Act., activation; IS, infectious spots; Intra, intracellular; Extra, extracellular; NO, no observed.

Nasal cytology: grid for semiquantitative analysis

	Microscopic field (immersion, ×1000)	o........ I........10 ....I........20......I........30......I........40......I........50				
	0 NO	+ (occasional)	++ (moderate)	+++ (many)	++++ (large number)	
Ciliated cells	0	20 20 20 20 20	20 20 20 20 20	20 20 20 20 20	20 20 20 20 20	SHS + % / CCP % / PNL %
Caliciform mucous cells	0	20 20 20 20 20	20 20 20 20 20	20 20 20 20 20	20 20 20 20 20	
Metaplasia	0	20 20 20 20 20	20 20 20 20 20	20 20 20 20 20	20 20 20 20 20	
Neutrophils	0	11 11 11 11 11 / 11 11 11 11 11	11 11 11 11 11 / 11 11 11 11 11	20 20 20	20 20 20	
Eosinophils	0	1 1 1 1 1	1 1 1 1 1	11 11 11 11 11 / 11 11 11 11 11	11 11 11 11 11 / 11 11 11 11 11	Degr. 0
Mast cells	0	1 1 1 1 1	1 1 1 1 1	11 11 11 11 11 / 11 11 11 11 11	11 11 11 11 11 / 11 11 11 11 11	Degr. 0
Lymphocytes	0	1 1 1 1 1	1 1 1 1 1	11 11 11 11 11 / 11 11 11 11 11	11 11 11 11 11 / 11 11 11 11 11	Act. %
Bacteria	0	I I I	II II	III III III	IIIIIIIIIIIIIIIIIIIII IIIIIIIIIIIIIIIIIIIII	Intra 0 / Extra 0
Spores	0	I I I	II II	III III III	IIIIIIIIIIIIIIIIIIIII IIIIIIIIIIIIIIIIIIIII	Hyphae 0 / IS 0

a

Nasal cytology: grid for semiquantitative analysis

	Microscopic field (immersion, ×1000)	o........ I........10 ....I........20......I........30......I........40......I........50				
	0 NO	+ (occasional)	++ (moderate)	+++ (many)	++++ (large number)	
Ciliated cells	⊠	20 20 20 20 20	20 20 20 20 20	20 20 20 20 20	20 20 20 20	
Caliciform mucous cells	0	2̶0̶ 2̶0̶ 2̶0̶ 20 20	20 20 20 20 20	20 20 20 20 20	20 20 20 2̶0̶	
Metaplasia	0	2̶0̶ 2̶0̶ 2̶0̶ 2̶0̶ 2̶0̶	2̶0̶ 2̶0̶ 2̶0̶ 2̶0̶ 2̶0̶	2̶0̶ 2̶0̶ 2̶0̶ 20 20	20 20 20 2̶0̶	
Neutrophils	⊠	11 11 11 11 11 / 11 11 11 11 11	11 11 11 11 11 / 11 11 11 11 11	20 20 20	20 20 20	
Eosinophils	0	✕ ✕ ✕ ✕ ✕	✕ ✕ ✕ ✕ ✕	✕ ✕ ✕ ✕ ✕ / ✕ ✕ ✕ ✕ ✕	✕ ✕ ✕ ✕ ✕ / ✕ ✕ ✕ ✕ ✕	Degr. ✕0
Mast cells	0	✕ ✕ ✕ ✕ ✕	✕ ✕ ✕ ✕ ✕	✕ ✕ ✕ ✕ ✕ / ✕ ✕ ✕ 11 11	11 11 11 11 11 / 11 11 11 11 11	Degr. ✕0
Lymphocytes	⊠	1 1 1 1 1	1 1 1 1 1	11 11 11 11 11 / 11 11 11 11 11	11 11 11 11 11 / 11 11 11 11 11	Act. %
Bacteria	⊠	I I I	II II	III III III	IIIIIIIIIIIIIIIIIIIII IIIIIIIIIIIIIIIIIIIII	Intra 0 / Extra 0
Spores	⊠	I I I	II II	III III III	IIIIIIIIIIIIIIIIIIIII IIIIIIIIIIIIIIIIIIIII	Hyphae 0 / IS 0

b

NASAL CYTOLOGY REPORT

Mr **John Brown**:
Number of fields examined at ×1000: 50.
No ciliated cells, rare mucous cells, numerous metaplastic cells.
No neutrophils, abundamt eosinophils, numerous mast cells, partly degranulated.
No lymphocytes, bacteria or spores.

c

Figure 6.26 Cell-counting grid. SHS, supranuclear hypercromatic striae; CCP, ciliocytophthoria; PNL, poynucleation; Degr., degranulation; Act., activation; IS, infectious spot; Intra, intracellular; Extra, extracellular. The operator should indicate, in the appropriate grid, the cytoype observed microscopically. This procedure will ensure a faster and easier cell counting relative to 50 microscopic fields at 1,000 magnification (**a**). The report will be prepared according to the cytotypes observed (**b**). Example of a report (**c**).

Nasal Cytopathology

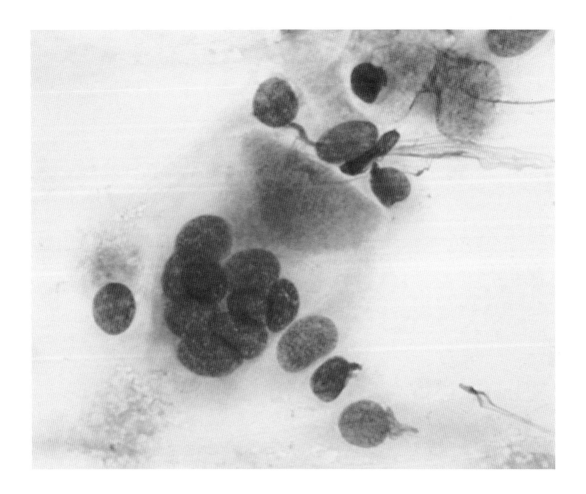

Making unjustified speculations and hypotheses is our only way to interpret nature. Those who refuse to state their ideas for fear of being disproved are not really playing the 'game of science'.

Karl Popper, 1934

Abnormal Cell Processes

An appreciation of the basic concepts of cytopathology is crucial to understanding the cytologic alterations that accompany nasal diseases.

Such alterations include degenerative, inflammatory, regenerative and neoplastic processes. Neoplastic alterations rarely occur in the nose and therefore fall outside the scope of this atlas. Readers interested in the latter are referred to the relevant literature published elsewhere.

DEGENERATIVE PROCESSES

The epithelial cells of the nasal mucosa, when exposed to insults of varying intensity and duration by various agents, undergo degeneration, frequently irreversible, leading to morphologic-volumetric changes involving the entire cell or a specific cell component (nucleus, cytoplasm, ciliary apparatus, etc.).

Nuclear alterations include:

- dyschromia
- pyknosis
- karyorrhexis
- karyolysis.

Nuclear *dyschromia* is an abnormality of the nuclear envelope (indistinct, discontinuous border) and the inner part of the nucleus (homogeneous appearance) where euchromatin cannot be distinguished from heterochromatin (**Fig. 7.1**).

Nuclear pyknosis is a destructive process in which the nucleus appears small and hyperchromatic (**Fig. 7.2**); it often results in cell senescence.

Nuclear karyorrhexis is fragmentation of the nucleus (**Fig. 7.3 a-b**) usually preceeded by gradual dyschromia, leading to karyolysis and enucleation (**Fig. 7.4 a-b**).

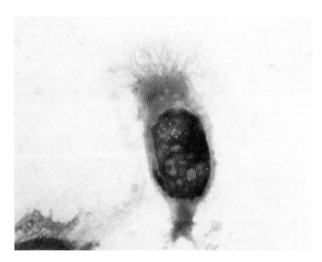

Figure 7.1 Nuclear dyschromia (MGG staining; ×1000).

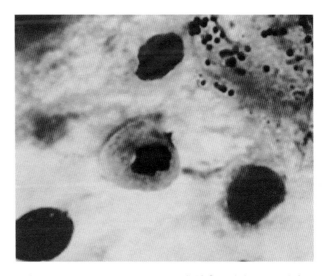

Figure 7.2 Nuclear pyknosis (MGG staining; ×1000).

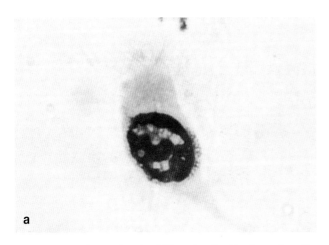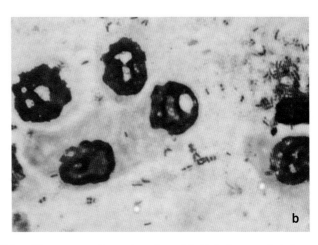

a b

Figure 7.3 Karyorrhexis. Ciliated cell with clear alteration of the ciliary apparatus and nucleus (**a**). Cell changes in infectious rhinitis. Elements of the Diplococcus genus and diphtheroids are clearly recognizable (**b**). MGG staining; ×1000.

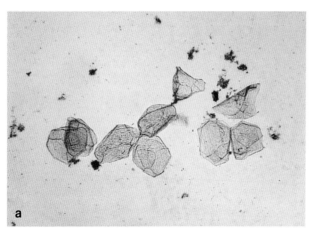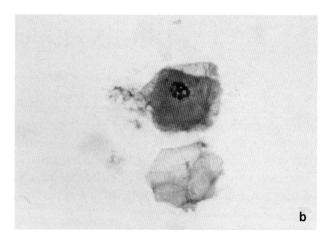

Figure 7.4 a-b Karyolysis. Cells of the nasal vestibule. The nucleus is not visible. The epithelial cells have a typical polygonal appearance (MGG staining; ×1000).

INFLAMMATORY PROCESSES

Finding occasional neutrophilic granulocytes on a nasal cytogram is not necessarily indicative of inflammation. In low numbers, these cells constitute the normal pool of phagocytes needed for ridding the respiratory nasal mucosa of invading pathogens.

By contrast, an elevated number of neutrophils is often associated with inflammatory processes: in this case, cell changes, often irreversible, take the form of non specific cytopathies and, less frequently, as for example in the case of invasion by certain microorganisms, characteristic features.

Non specific inflammatory processes include:
- nuclear swelling (**Fig. 7.5**);
- binucleation (**Fig. 7.6**);
- hyperchromia with margination of nuclear chromatin (**Fig. 7.7**);
- prominent nucleoli (**Fig. 7.8**);
- cytoplasmic vacuolization (**Fig. 7.9**).

In a setting of microbial infection, an elevated number of bacteria is associated with increased neutrophilic granulocytes. Bacteria and/or intracellular inclusions in the cytoplasm of neutrophilic granulocytes is a typical expression of phagocytosis (**Fig. 7.10**).

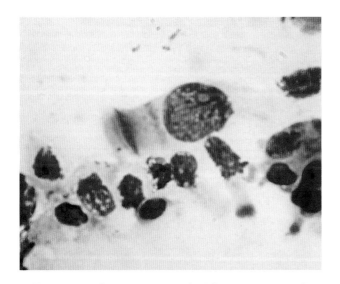

Figure 7.5 Swollen nucleus (MGG staining; ×1000).

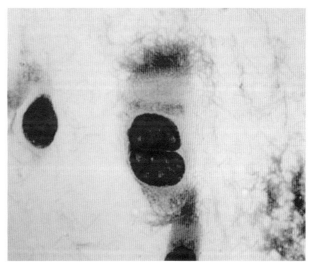

Figure 7.6 Binucleation (MGG staining; ×1000).

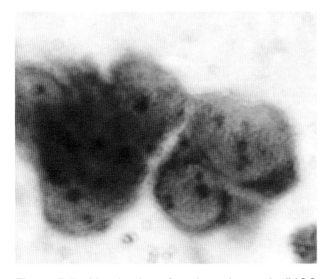

Figure 7.7 Margination of nuclear chromatin (MGG staining; ×1000 with CMF 4×).

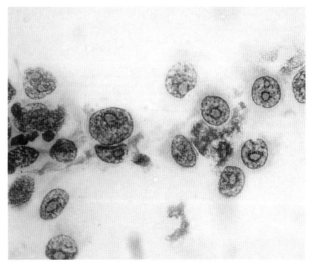

Figure 7.8 Prominent nucleoli (MGG staining; ×1000 with CMF 1.2×).

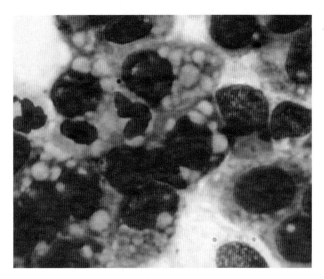

Figure 7.9 Cytoplasmic vacuolization (MGG staining; ×1000 with CMF 2.2×).

In viral infections, cells may demonstrate multi-nucleation and ciliocytophthoria.

Infected cells may contain a variable number of nuclei with a typical ground glass appearance that prevents detailed observation of the chromatin. Large dark red intranuclear inclusions may also be present.

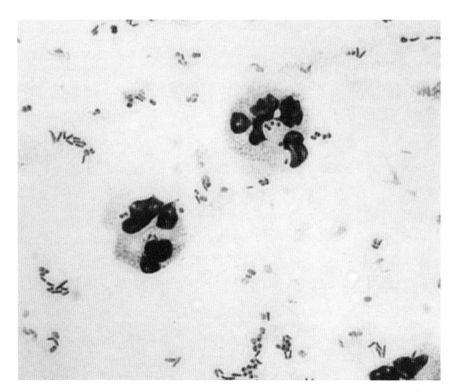

Figure 7.10 Bacterial rhinitis. Extracellular and intracellular bacteria inside the neutrophils (MGG staining; ×1000 with CMF 2.2×).

REPAIR PROCESSES

There exist characteristic features of repair processes following episodes of inflammation, infection and trauma, including post-surgical ones, that should not be confused with degenerative changes (dyskaryosis, etc.).

A typical expression of repair is cell aggregation (**Fig. 7.11 a**) in which the cells may appear polynucleate with no more than 4-5 nuclei (**Fig. 7.11 b**) and with prominent nucleoli. Polynucleation is a frequent finding. The distinguishing feature is that the nuclei maintain their finely granular chromatin structure.

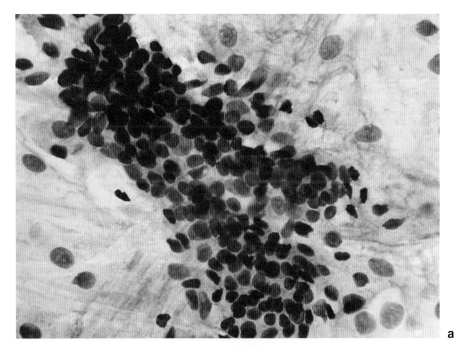

a

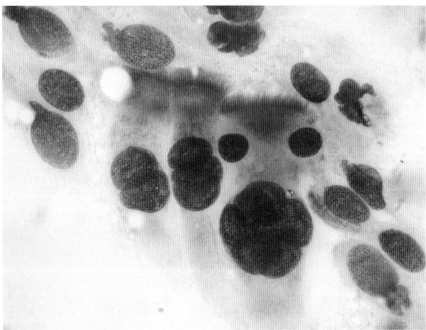

b

Figure 7.11 Cell cluster (**a**); ciliated cells showing polynucleation (**b**). MGG staining; **a**, ×1000; **b**, ×1000 with CMF 1.4×).

CYTOLOGIC FINDINGS IN NASAL DISEASES

In healthy children and adults, the nasal mucosa is composed of numerous epithelial cells: ciliated cells, striate cells, goblet cells and basal cells. In the superficial epithelial layer of the basement membrane, eosinophils and mast cells are usually absent, while a cytologic sample from the anterior portion of the inferior turbinate may include sporadic neutrophils and bacteria.

In pathologic conditions (**Fig. 7.12**), the cellular component of the nasal mucosa is altered, leading to the appearance of certain cell types usually absent in normal mucosa.

These changes make cytologic examination a useful aid in establishing the correct diagnosis, monitoring the course of the disease, and evaluating response to pharmacologic therapy.

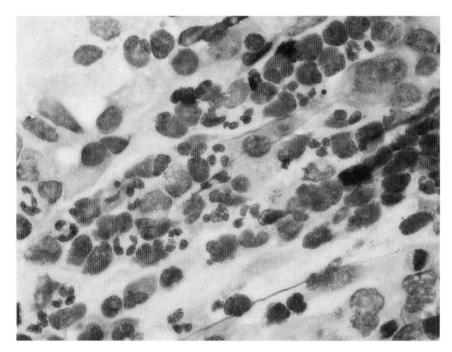

Figure 7.12   Acute allergic rhinitis. Eosinophils, neutrophils, lymphocytes and mast cells are clearly present (MGG staining; ×1000).

CLASSIFICATION OF RHINITIS

The recent ARIA (*Allergic Rhinitis and its Impact on Asthma*) 2011 guidelines report my newly proposed and more complete classification of rhinopathologies, which includes descriptions, of the "non allergic" vasomotor forms, and of nasal diseases with a "cellular" expression. It also includes well codified nosological entities of which the most recently described is non allergic rhinitis with eosinophils and mast cells (NARESMA) (**Fig. 7.13**).

RHINOPATHIES	Infectious	Acute Chronic	Viral Bacterial Fungal	
	Inflammatory	Physicochemical-environmental agents		
	Vasomotor	Allergic	Intermittent (previously defined seasonal) Persistent (previously defined perennial)	
		Non allergic ("cellular")	Neutrophilic (NARNE) Eosinophilic (NARES) With mast cells (NARMA) Eosinophilic with mast cells (NARESMA)	
	Hyperplastic/ granulomatous	Nasal polyposis - Antrochoanal polyp - Wegener's granulomatosis - Sarcoidosis - Churg-Strauss syndrome		
	Neoplasia	Inverted papilloma - Fibroma - Chondroma - Angioma - Carcinoma - Sarcoma, etc.		
	Atrophic	Senile or induced by chronic rhinitis processes		
	Iatrogenic	Induced by overuse of α-adrenergics, α-blockers, cocaine, clonidine, ACE inhibitors, oral contraceptives, antiepileptic drugs, antipsychotics, aspirin and other NSAIDs, calcium channel blockers		
	Hormonal	Hypothyroidism-related Pregnancy-related Premenstrual		
	Others	Adrenergic or antispastic - Cholinergic Gustatory (oronasal syndrome) Mechanical (septal deviation, foreign bodies, choanal atresia, adenoids, etc.) Decubitus-induced – Induced by physical exercise Occupational (allergic and non allergic) Psychotic-emotional - Sexual arousal Ciliary dyskinesia – Cystic fibrosis – Meningoencephalocele		

Figure 7.13 Gelardi's classification of rhinopathies as accepted by the Commission for ARIA (*Allergic Rhinitis and its Impact on Asthma*) 2011 guidelines. This text deals only with those in which diagnostic cytology plays an important role: infectious rhinitis (bacterial, viral, and fungal forms), inflammatory rhinitis, vasomotor rhinitis (allergic and non allergic), hyperplastic/granulomatous (nasal polyposis) and atrophic rhinitis.
NARNE (non allergic rhinitis with neutrophils); NARES (non allergic rhinitis with eosinophilia syndrome); NARMA (non allergic rhinitis with mast cells); NARESMA (non allergic rhinitis with eosinophils and mast cells).

Nasal Cytopathology – INFECTIOUS RHINITIS

INFECTIOUS RHINITIS

Bacterial Rhinitis

In the presence of inflammation, a variety of resident or circulating cell populations (neutrophils, lymphocytes, macrophages) may appear on the surface of the respiratory mucosa, raising the number of exfoliated epithelial cells, the majority of which show alterations.

In addition to numerous neutrophils, microscopic observation will reveal other microbes: bacteria bound to the cell surface and bacteria inside phagocytes (macrophages and neutrophils) (**Figs. 7.14** to **7.23**).

Furthermore, the presence of bacteria and neu-

trophils is associated with the following cytologic abnormalities:

- reduced number of ciliated cells;
- increased number of goblet cells, metaplastic and squamous cells;
- increased number of lymphocytes, macrophages and plasma cells;
- the presence of an infectious spot, the morphologic-chromatic expression of biofilm (**Figs. 7.24-7.25**).

During the course of medical treatment, cytologic studies should be performed regularly to

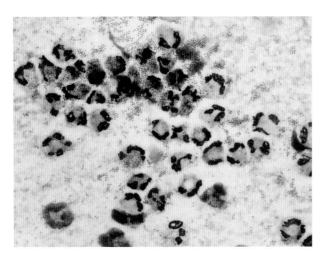

Figure 7.14 Bacterial rhinitis. Numerous neutrophils and bacteria in nasal secretion (MGG staining; ×1000).

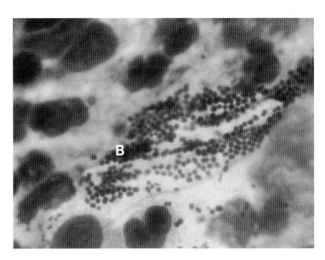

Figure 7.15 Bacterial rhinitis. Bacterial colony (B). At the center of the bacterial colony it is possible to detect a faint "cyan" color, which is the expression of an initial biofilm formation (MGG staining; ×1000 with CMF 1.2×).

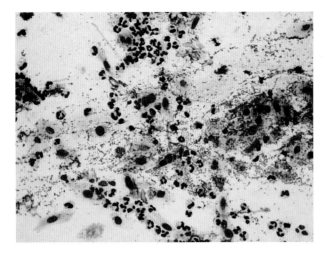

Figure 7.16 Bacterial rhinitis. Numerous neutrophils and bacteria in nasal secretion (MGG staining; ×400).

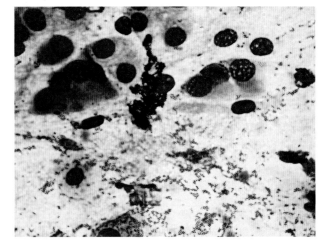

Figure 7.17 Bacterial rhinitis. Numerous bacteria and metaplastic cells in nasal secretion (MGG staining; ×1000).

Atlas of NASAL CYTOLOGY for the Differential Diagnosis of Nasal Diseases

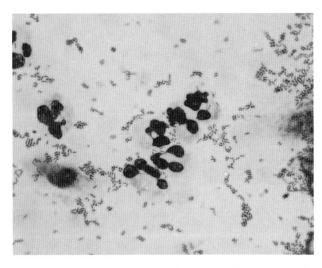

Figure 7.18 Bacterial rhinitis. Sporadic neutrophils and numerous bacteria (MGG staining; ×1000 with CMF 2.2×).

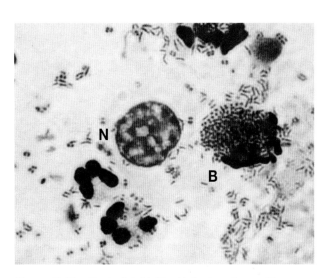

Figure 7.19 Bacterial rhinitis. Naked nucleus with prominent nucleolus (N), bacterial colony (B) (MGG staining; ×1000 with CMF 2.4×).

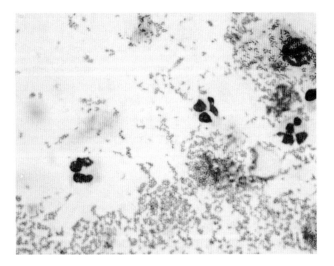

Figure 7.20 Bacterial rhinitis. Sporadic neutrophils and numerous bacteria (MGG staining; ×1000).

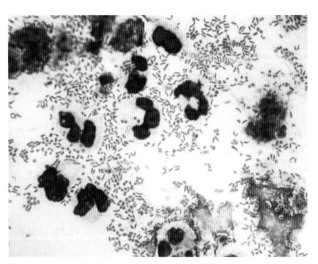

Figure 7.21 Bacterial rhinitis. Sporadic neutrophils and numerous bacteria (MGG staining; ×1000 with CMF 2.2×).

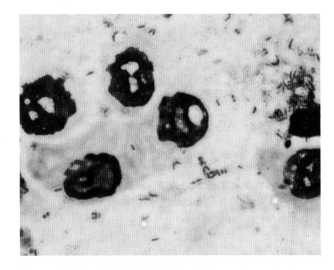

Figure 7.22 Bacterial rhinitis. Cells undergoing karyorrhexis and bacteria (MGG staining; ×1000 with CMF 2.4×).

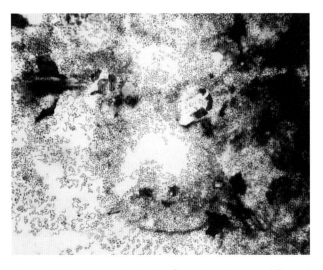

Figure 7.23 Bacterial rhinitis. Occasional neutrophils and numerous bacteria (MGG staining; ×1000).

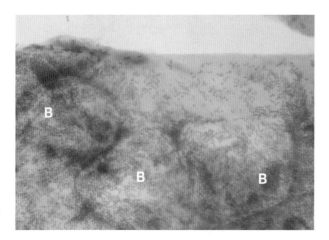

Figure 7.24 Bacterial rhinitis: cyan-colored infectious spots, the morphologic-chromatic expression of biofilm. Numerous bacteria (B) embedded in the exopolysaccharide matrix (MGG staining; ×1000).

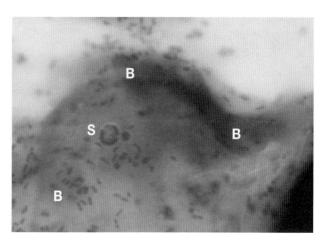

Figure 7.25 Bacterial rhinitis: cyan-colored infectious spots, the morphologic-chromatic expression of biofilm. Numerous bacteria (B) and spores (S) embedded in the exopolysaccharide matrix (MGG staining; ×1000 with CMF 1.2×).

monitor these forms of rhinitis. Only after a major reduction in the number of inflammatory cells and the nearly complete clearance of bacteria from the cytologic sample can resolution of the disease be confirmed.

Viral Infectious Rhinitis

Acute respiratory infection is commonly caused by a virus (**Table 7.1**), even though the viral infection often leads to an overlapping bacterial infection, favored in part by the cytopathic effect of the virus on the mucosal epithelium.

The most common viruses found in the respiratory tract are:
- myxoviruses (influenza viruses)
- paramyxovirus (parainfluenza viruses)
- respiratory syncytial virus (RSV)
- picornaviruses (Coxsackie A and B viruses, enteric viruses and ECHO [*enteric cytopathic human orphan*] viruses)
- adenoviruses
- herpes virus (serotype 1).

Table 7.1 Common viruses causing respiratory infections

RNA viruses	rhinoviruses	25-30%
	myxoviruses	10-15%
	coronaviruses	8-10%
	enteric viruses	5%
DNA viruses	adenoviruses	5%
Unidentified viruses		30-35%

In viral infections, the nasal mucosa appears congested, edematous and covered with a seromucous exudate.

Microscopic observation reveals respiratory mucosal damage primarily involving the superficial epithelium. The epithelial cells are lysed by viruses and cytotoxic T lymphocytes, whereas, unlike what occurs in bacterial infection, the subepithelial structures show only moderate damage.

Superficial epithelial regeneration takes place through exchange cells, with complete healing at the end of the viral episode. This is in contrast to what occurs in bacterial infection, where the bacteria disrupt the basement membrane and vessel of the *tunica propria*, often leaving scars.

Studies on the cellular infiltrate found in nasal mucosa after viral infection have shown that the number of polymorphonuclear leukocytes increases within 24 hours of viral invasion and that the infiltration by neutrophils is accompanied by increased numbers of lymphocytes and exfoliated epithelial cells.

Lymphocytes are predominant whereas leukocytes are predominant in bacterial superinfection. In bacterial superinfection, the mucosal surface is covered with an exudate of variable purulent composition, which is the expression of the passage of neutrophils to the surface.

As in other epithelia, viral infections in the respiratory epithelium can produce characteristic cytopathologic effects, depending on the virus in question.

During the first week of infection, rhinoviruses and coronaviruses provoke no specific damage to the nasal mucosa. The ciliated cells preserve their normal ciliary beat and remain compact. This has been confirmed in histopathologic studies showing

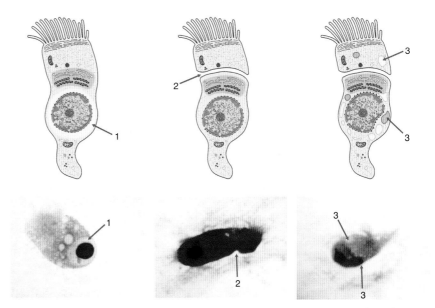

Figure 7.26 Signs of viral cytopathology (ciliocytopthoria):
1. perinuclear halo;
2. separation of basal nucleus-containing portion from the ciliated apical portion;
3. cytoplasmic granules and inclusion bodies.

that only 2% of respiratory mucosal cells test positive to the rhinovirus antigen and that replication is positive only in some cells even during major manifestation of clinical symptoms.

By contrast, influenza viruses and adenoviruses destroy the epithelial cells during the initial period of infection.

Respiratory syncytial virus (RSV) is responsible for cytopathologic effects by the fourth day of infection, with cytolysis occurring on the seventh day.

With the exception of forms caused by influenza viruses and adenoviruses, this evidence runs counter to the old idea that cold symptoms result from the destruction of the nasal mucosal epithelium. Further evidence that mucosal damage does not commonly cause cold symptoms is the fact that rhinoviruses and coronaviruses, which are known to be less aggressive, are the most common causal agents of "influenza" symptoms.

The ciliated epithelia undergo morphologic changes encompassed by the term *ciliocytophthoria*. Classically, these alterations include nuclear chromatin condensation, nuclear margination, the appearance of inclusions (inclusion bodies), halo formation around the nucleus, the appearance of cytoplasmic granules, constriction of the cell body, and separation of the basal nucleus-containing portion from the ciliated apical portion (**Fig. 7.26**). Our studies, still ongoing, suggest morphologic interpretations other than ciliocytophthoria. In particular, the change commonly described as a "perinuclear" halo is actually just an intranuclear area devoid of chromatin. This is confirmed by the constant presence of rounded formations probably representing nucleoli.

Other cytopathologic effects are nuclear alterations (typical ground glass appearance), syncytial features and inclusion bodies.

In herpes virus infection, we have found alterations involving ciliated columnar cells and mucous cells. These changes lead to a considerable increase in cell volume associated with polynucleation (**Figs. 7.27-7.29**).

Viral infection was confirmed at electron microscopy which allowed identification of the virus (**Fig. 7.30**).

In the same cytologic preparations we also found cells with spherical intracytoplasmic inclusions that stained dark red-fuchsia with MGG (**Figs. 7.31-7.33**). Later PAS staining, which is selective for mucopolysaccharides, revealed that the inclusion was a collection of mucus.

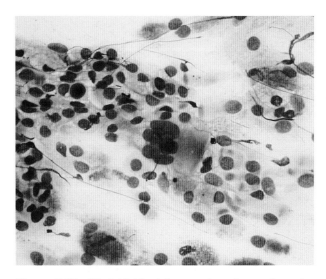

Figure 7.27 Viral rhinitis. A large polynuclear cell can be seen in the center of the field (MGG staining; ×400).

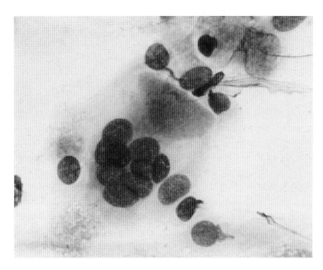

Figure 7.28 Viral rhinitis. A large polynuclear cell at higher magnification (MGG staining; ×1000 with CMF 2.0×).

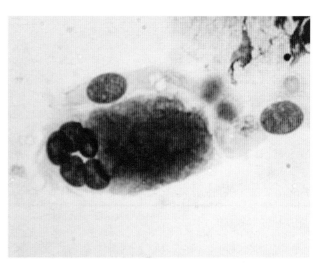

Figure 7.29 Viral rhinitis. Polynucleation can also involve mucous cells (MGG staining; ×1000 with CMF 2.0×).

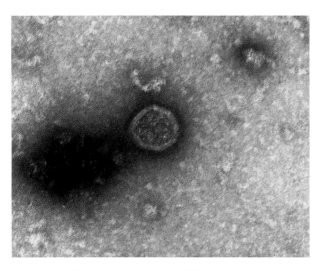

Figure 7.30 Herpes virus (Electron microscopy ×63,000).

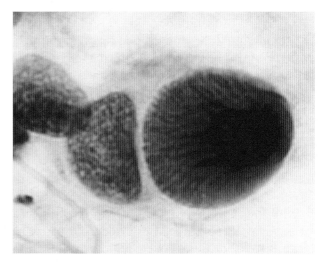

Figure 7.31 Viral rhinitis. Detailed view of morphologic and staining characteristics of a secretory cell (MGG staining; ×1000 with CMF 4.0×).

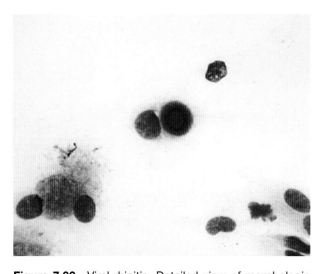

Figure 7.32 Viral rhinitis. Detailed view of morphologic and staining characteristics of a secretory cell (MGG staining; ×1000).

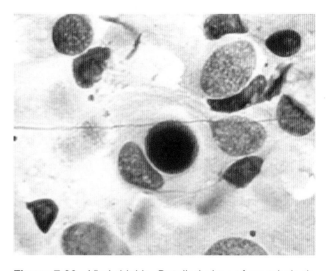

Figure 7.33 Viral rhinitis. Detailed view of morphologic and staining characteristics of a secretory cell (MGG staining; ×1000 with CMF 1.2×).

In viral infections, after an initial marked drop in the number of ciliated cells, which is the primary cause of alterations in mucociliary clearance, there is a gradual regeneration of the cilia. The more rapidly mucociliary clearance is restored, the lower the risk of bacterial complications.

Fungal Rhinitis

The airways are a readily available site for fungal infection because spores – ubiquitous in nature and highly resistant to atmospheric agents – can easily reach the anatomic structures of the airway surface which are in direct contact by air. The nasal fossae are rarely affected by common fungi (candida, *Aspergillus*, *Penicillum*). In immunocompromised subjects, however, the nose may be a site of severe primary infection (rhinosporidosis, rhinocerebral zygomycosis).

Depending on the etiologic agent involved, the infection may be endogenous or exogenous and lead to deep, subcutaneous or superficial manifestations, involving the skin, the cutaneous adnexa or the mucosa. The name given an entity is usually derived from the anatomic structure affected (e.g. dermatomycosis, onychomycosis, otomycosis) or more often from the name of the fungus (aspergillosis, candidiasis, sporotrichosis, etc.).

Clinical manifestations develop in relation to patient-related factors (age, carbohydrate-rich or vitamin-poor diet) or disease-related factors (immune deficiencies, metabolic disorders, prolonged corticosteroid pharmacologic therapy). Alterations in the body's response to fungal invasion may range from mild antibody production to specific hypersensitivity reactions.

In most anatomic areas, the clinical picture of fungal infection is diagnostic (e.g. serous and serofibrinous infection can often be found in lesions of the oral mucosa; thrush is caused by candida yeasts). By contrast, pathognomonic manifestations are rarely observed in the nasal mucosa where the insidious course of infection makes diagnosis difficult without the aid of cytologic and microbiologic studies.

Catarrhal forms are generally caused by yeasts, aspergilli, actinomycetes, and zygomycetes, all of which can produce purulent inflammation.

In all sites of infection (skin, mucosa, etc.), fungi can sensitize the host even in the absence of specific symptoms. In these cases, the diagnosis can be established on the basis of skin allergy tests. An intradermal response that is positive to a fungal extract is the expression of an active or previous infection. The intradermal response can be positive even years after clinical resolution of the infection. In this way, a fungal cause of allergic manifestations, such as rhinitis, asthma, urticaria and dermatitis, can be demonstrated. For several years now there has been debate on the possible fungal causes of some forms of nasal polyposis, but to date there is no scientific evidence to confirm this hypothesis. By contrast, some fungi may be responsible for severe sinus diseases, as in the case of invasive fungal rhinosinusitis, and for less severe forms, such as "fungus balls".

An understanding of the allergenic properties of fungi is important in the case of occupational fungal allergies observed in agricultural or industrial workers. Sources of allergenic fungi (**Table 7.2**) include soils (for *Penicillium*, *Aspergillus*, *Alternaria*, *Cladosporium*, *Mucorales*, etc.); decomposing vegetation; edible fruits and vegetables (for *Penicillum*, *Trichothecium*, etc.); and textile fibers such as cotton, wool, linen, hemp fabrics (for *Penicillium*, *Aspergillus*, *Fusarium*, *Cladosporium*, etc.).

Airborne spore levels are influenced by a host of factors: temperature, humidity, wind, changing of the seasons and changes in the weather.

Although allergenic fungi are more prevalent in certain seasons, the presence of fungi does not vary in general, except for *Cladosporium*, which are most frequent in winter, and *Alternaria* which peak in late spring and summer.

Alternaria species is thought to be primarily responsible for causing asthma and have been isolated in individuals affected by the condition.

Cultures are indispensable for determining the causal agent because they permit identification of the fungal species or can rule out commensal agents. In many cases, the presence of mixed infections (bacterial and fungal) should be investigated, since they are a common side effect of local or systemic antibiotic or corticosteroid therapy.

Table 7.2 Fungal species

• *Alternaria*	• *Helminthosporium*
• *Aspergillus*	• *Mucor*
• *Cladosporium*	• *Penicillium*
• *Curvalaria*	• *Pullularia*
• *Epicoccum*	• *Stemphyllium*
• *Fusarium*	

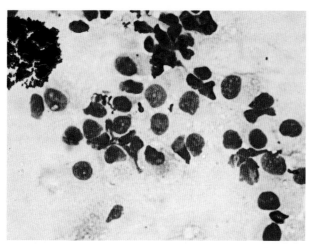

Figure 7.34 Fungal rhinitis. Several fungal spores can be seen in the center of the field. In fungal infections, nuclear alterations can vary from rarefaction to karyorrhexis (MGG staining; ×1000).

The cytopathologic effects of fungi manifest chiefly in the nuclei, producing characteristic nuclear rarefaction. Another possible finding is intracellular invasion (cytoplasm and nucleus) by spores or fungal hyphae (**Figs. 7.34, 7.35 a-d**).

To correctly diagnose these diseases, it is paramount to know the cytopathologies. Since they are readily visible even at medium-power magnification (×400), these are features that can be confirmed with high-power magnification (immersion ×1000).

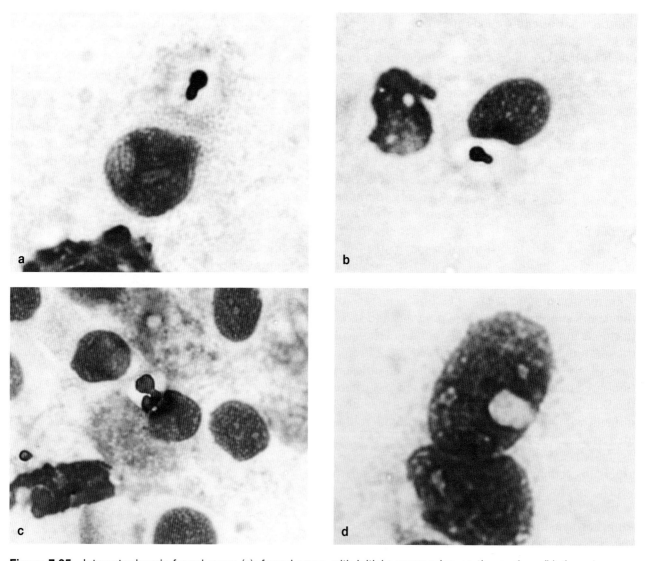

Figure 7.35 Intracytoplasmic fungal spore (**a**); fungal spore with initial compression on the nucleus (**b**); fungal spores compressing the nucleus, with prominent chromatin condensation at the pressure point (**c**); "chewed" appearance of the nucleus (**d**) (MGG staining; ×1000; **a-c**, CMF 3×; **d**, CMF 4×).

INFLAMMATORY RHINITIS

Long-term exposure to airborne irritants (atmospheric pollutants, tobacco smoke) initiates chronic inflammation that disrupts the mucosal integrity of the upper airways (nose, nasopharynx and larynx) and the pulmonary parenchyma (**Fig. 7.36**). This is exacerbated by gradual destruction of mucosal tissue.

Reduced mucociliary clearance, resulting from ciliary dyskinesia caused by irritants and inflammation-induced changes, promotes bacterial colonization, leading to infection.

Subsequently, chronic inflammation worsens as tissues are destroyed or remodeled, leading to further impairment of the defense mechanisms of the superficial tissue layers.

A similar process is initiated by congenital disorders characterized by mucociliary clearance dysfunctions, including primary ciliary dyskinesia syndrome, secretory IgA deficiency, and mucoviscidosis (cystic fibrosis), all of which are particularly insidious in their severe forms.

In healthy individuals with intact airways, the likelihood that single episodes of viral and/or bacterial infection will give rise to chronic inflammation is low, except in cases of local anatomic obstruction (paranasal and middle ear obstructions) where even moderate epithelial damage may lead to recurrence of the disorder. Alterations of the respiratory epithelium following tissue damage, which are associated with abnormal tissue remodeling, manifest as areas of muciparous or platycellular metaplasia (**Fig. 7.37**).

In heavy smokers and individuals chronically exposed to airborne pollutants, numerous changes in the number and character of respiratory epithelial cells have been described. These include intense exfoliation with anomalous morphology of individual cells (squat or spherical), cells fused in pairs or triads with shortened, disorderly or twisted cilia, and swollen nuclei. In workers exposed to extreme work environments (large temperature excursions, industrial vapors and dusts) there may also be an elevated number of goblet cells (muciparous prevalence).

The effect of exposure to intranasal stimuli has been studied in nasal cytology (**Table 7.3**).

Stimulation with saline or distilled water provokes no change in the number or type of cells found in the nasal lavage fluid, whereas exposure to formaldehyde can cause epithelial metaplasia

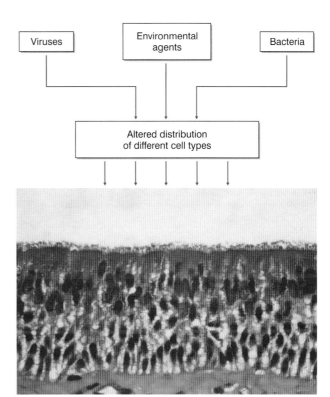

Figure 7.36 Principal agents of change in the respiratory epithelium.

Table 7.3 Nasal cytology and exposure to physicochemical stimuli

Stimulus	Effect
Cold water	No cell change
Distilled water	No cell change
Saline solution	No cell change
Formaldehyde	Occasional platycellular/muciparous metaplasia
Cigarette smoking	Occasional platycellular/muciparous metaplasia (depending on number of pack-years)
α-adrenergics	No cell change

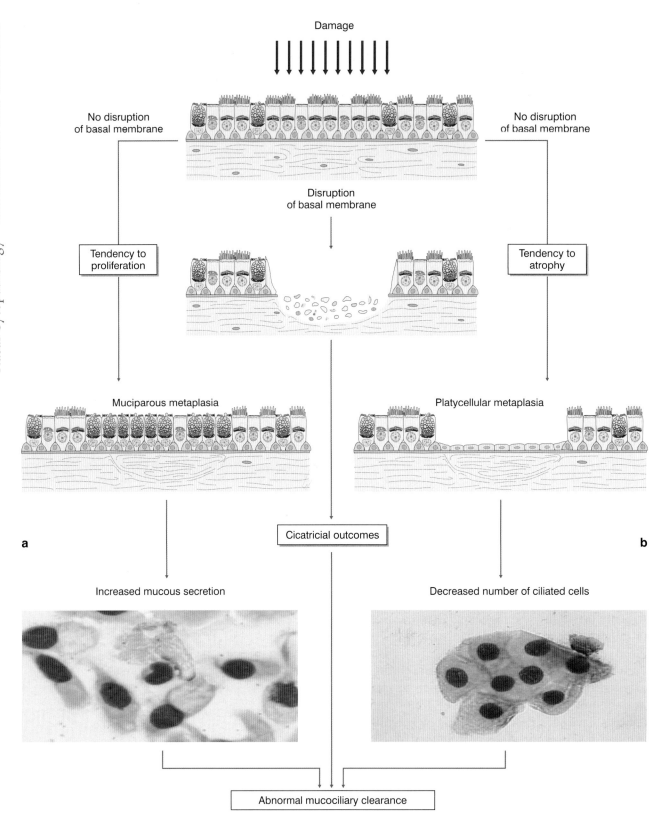

Damage

No disruption
of basal membrane

No disruption
of basal membrane

Tendency to
proliferation

Disruption
of basal membrane

Tendency to
atrophy

Muciparous metaplasia

Platycellular metaplasia

a

Cicatricial outcomes

b

Increased mucous secretion

Decreased number of ciliated cells

Abnormal mucociliary clearance

Figure 7.37 Principal agents of change in the respiratory epithelium. In chronic inflammation is that the epithelium may gradually undergo metaplasia, tending toward either the proliferating form in which the number of goblet cells increases (muciparous metaplasia, **a**), or the atrophic form with an increased number of squamous cells (platycellular metaplasia, **b**). The atrophic forms occur more often in older persons, while younger persons are more subject to proliferating metaplasia.

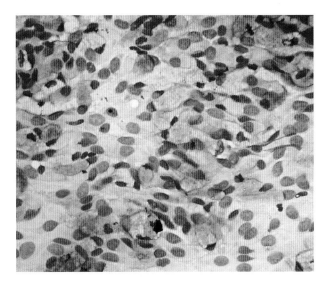

Figure 7.38 Muciparous metaplasia (MGG staining; ×1000).

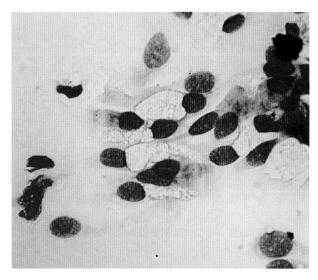

Figure 7.39 Muciparous metaplasia. Goblet cells outnumber ciliated cells (MGG staining; ×1000 with CMF 1×).

and dysplasia. Cigarette smoking causes metaplasia and often dysplasia, depending on the number of pack-years.

Exposure to cold air produces no changes in the number or type of cells. α-adrenergic agents may cause rhinitis medicamentosa, without evidence of cell changes.

What is important in chronic inflammation is that the epithelium may gradually undergo meta-plasia, tending toward either the proliferating form in which the number of goblet cells increases (muciparous metaplasia) (**Figs. 7.38-7.40**), or the atrophic form with an increased number of squamous cells (platycellular metaplasia) (**Figs. 7.40, 7.41**). The atrophic forms occur more often in older persons, while younger persons are more subject to proliferating metaplasia.

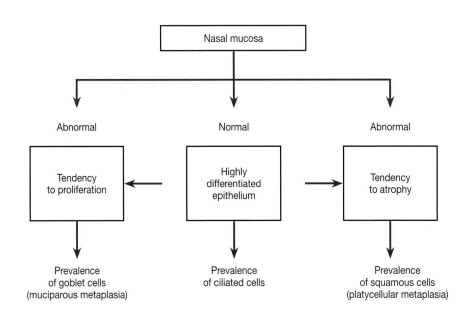

Figure 7.40 Changes in the epithelium of the nasal mucosa in chronic inflammation.

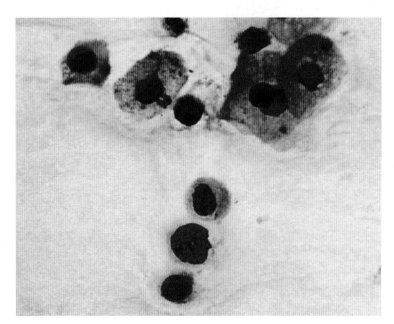

Figure 7.41 Platycellular metaplasia (MGG staining; ×1000).

VASOMOTOR RHINITIS

Vasomotor rhinitis is a large category that includes "allergic" and "non allergic" forms (**Fig. 7.13**).

Allergic Rhinitis

In patients with seasonal or perennial allergic rhinitis, natural or specific provocation produces an immediate (early phase) or delayed (late phase) response (**Fig. 7.42**). Microscopically, these responses are characterized by immuno-inflammatory infiltrations (eosinophils, mast cells, neutrophils and lymphocytes) (**Figs. 7.43, 7.45-7.63**) and by the presence of numerous chemical mediators in the nasal discharge. These chemical mediators are responsible for the main symptoms characterizing the condition (nasal itching and congestion, sneezing, rhinorrhea, tearing, etc.).

Long-term, low-intensity allergen exposure (dermatophagoides, *Parietaria*), as occurs in perennial rhinitis, leads to the development of *minimal persistent inflammation* (**Fig. 7.47**) characterized mainly by invasion of neutrophils and to a lesser extent by eosinophils and mast cells. These cells and the mediators they release produce the subchronic symptoms typical of perennial allergic rhinitis.

A non allergic individual showing no response to the nasal provocation test (**Fig. 7.44 a-b**) will not demonstrate any cell changes on the nasal cytogram. By contrast, individuals with specific allergies will demonstrate significant changes in inflammatory cells of the sub- and supraepithelial layers, with increased numbers of neutrophils, eosinophils and mononuclear cells. However they will not shown

differences in the proportion of cell types composing the nasal mucosa (goblet, striated and basal cells).

The remarkable feature is the chronologic sequence of cell types that emerge on the mucosal surface following antigen challenge (**Fig. 7.45**). The number of neutrophils begins to increase, peaking at 6 h post-challenge, and remains constant over the next 48 h. Eosinophils increase in number starting from 2 h post-challenge and peak at around 10 h, diminishing thereafter.

Mast cells are present to a lesser extent and their concentration is highest at 15 h post-challenge, after which it gradually decreases. The use of specific dyes will help distinguish the various cell types. *Toluidine blue* will stain the metachromatic granules of mast cells and basophils, but MGG staining is sufficient for the "trained" eye (**Figs. 7.53, 7.54**).

Generally, an increase in metachromatic cells is accompanied by worsening symptoms and a more marked response to the provocation test. By assessing these cells in addition to the eosinophils, the sensitivity of the cytologic test is enhanced, allowing confirmation of allergy.

Eosinophils can be found in allergic individuals of any age, whereas the presence of intra- and extracellular bacteria associated with numerous neutrophils

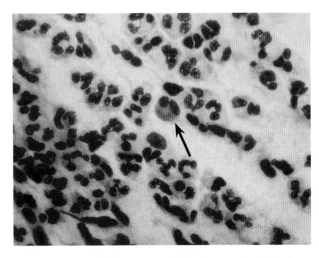

Figure 7.43 "Minimal persistent inflammation" is characterized by continued mild symptoms (nasal congestion, mild itching and rhinorrhea). The nasal cytogram shows numerous neutrophils, sporadic eosinophils and lymphocytes. At the center of the microscopic field there is an eosinophil (arrow) surrounded by numerous neutrophils (MGG staining; ×1000).

Figure 7.42 Immediate and delayed response to the nasal provocation test.

Stimulus

Immediate nasal response

Time (h) 0 1 2 3 4 5 6 7 8 9 10 11 12 13 14 15 16 17 18 19 20 21 22 23 24

Delayed nasal response

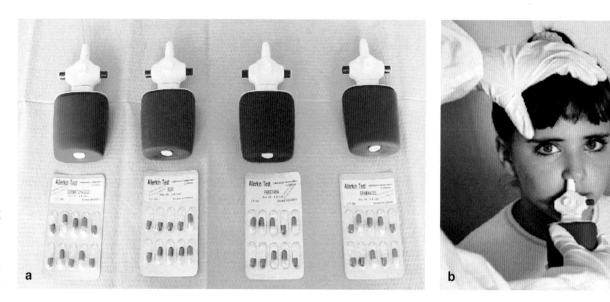

Figure 7.44 Nasal provocation test with Allerkin® (**a-b**).

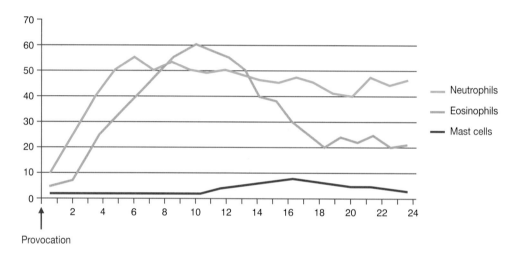

Figure 7.45 Cellularity after allergen-specific nasal provocation testing: changes in cell types after testing with Allerkin®.

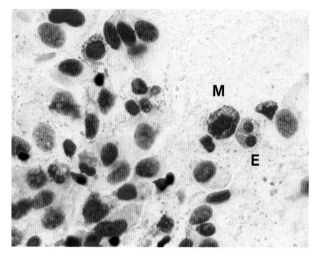

Figure 7.46 Allergic rhinitis. Eosinophil (E) and mast cell (M) (MGG staining; ×1000).

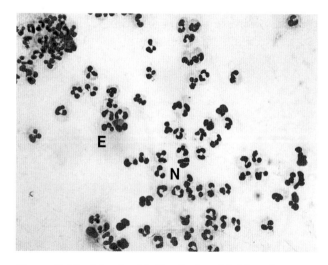

Figure 7.47 Allergic rhinitis. Eosinophil (E) and numerous neutrophils (N) ("minimal persistent inflammation") (MGG staining; ×400).

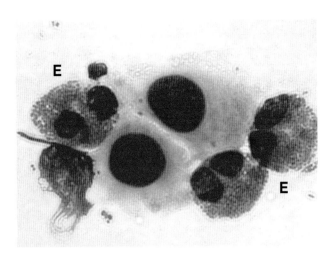

Figure 7.48 Allergic rhinitis. Eosinophils (E) (MGG staining; ×1000 with CMF 2.4×).

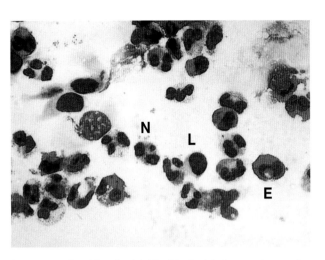

Figure 7.49 Allergic rhinitis. Typical inflammatory cells: neutrophils (N), eosinophils (E), lymphocytes (L) (MGG staining; ×1000).

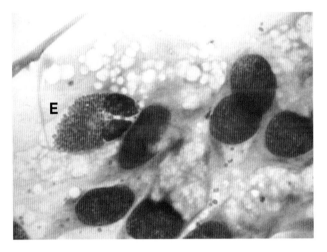

Figure 7.50 Allergic rhinitis. Eosinophil (E) demonstrating characteristic acidophilic staining of cytoplasmic granules and bilobated nucleus surrounded by goblet cells (MGG staining; ×1000 with CMF 2.4×).

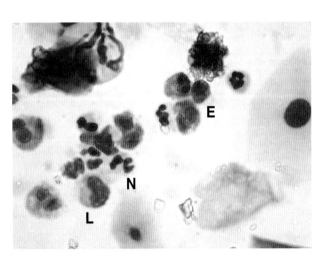

Figure 7.51 Allergic rhinitis. Typical inflammatory cells: neutrophils (N), eosinophils (E), lymphocytes (L); nasal lavage (MGG staining; ×1000).

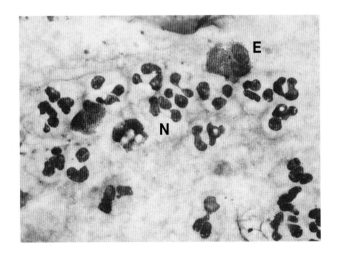

Figure 7.52 Allergic rhinitis. Characteristic reddish-orange staining of cytoplasmic granules permits discrimination between eosinophils (E) and neutrophils (N) (MGG staining; ×1000).

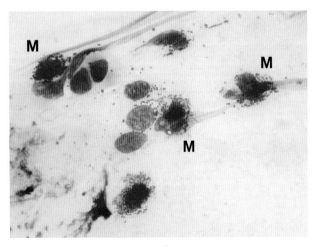

Figure 7.53 Allergic rhinitis. Group of degranulating mast cells (M) (MGG staining; ×1000).

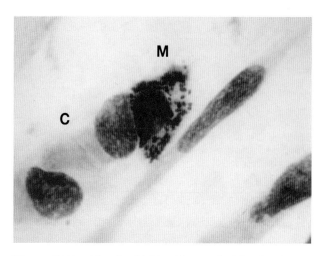

Figure 7.54 Allergic rhinitis. Mast cell (M) adhering to columnar cell (C) of the nasal epithelium (MGG staining; ×1000 with CMF 2.2×).

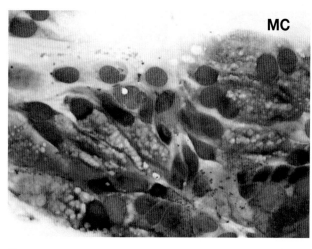

Figure 7.55 Allergic rhinitis. Prevalence of goblet cells is a consistent finding in allergic rhinitis. Muciparous cell (MC) with intracytoplasmic vacuoles (MGG staining; ×1000).

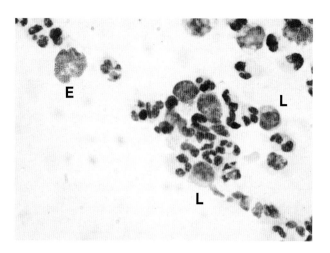

Figure 7.56 Allergic rhinitis. Presence of lymphocytes (L) is characteristic of allergic rhinitis. Eosinophils (E) (MGG staining; ×1000).

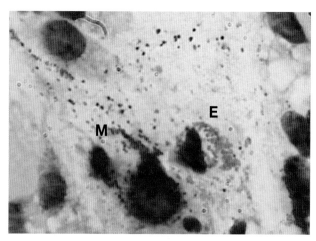

Figure 7.57 Allergic rhinitis. Degranulation. Specific dye affinity permits discrimination between cell types even when the cell has lost its morphologic characteristics. Eosinophil (E), mast cell (M) (MGG staining; ×1000 with CMF 2×).

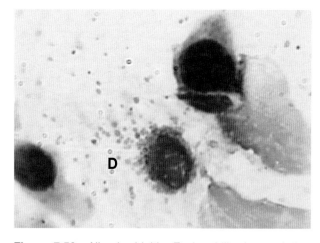

Figure 7.58 Allergic rhinitis. Eosinophilic degranulation (D) (MGG staining; ×1000 with CMF 1.4×).

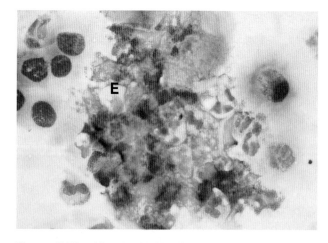

Figure 7.59 Allergic rhinitis. Degranulating eosinophils (E). The cells are unrecognizable but the staining characteristics of the granules covering nearly the entire microscopic field indicate they are eosinophils (MGG staining; ×1000).

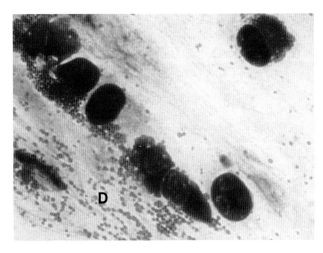

Figure 7.60 Allergic rhinitis. Eosinophilic degranulating (D) (MGG staining; ×1000).

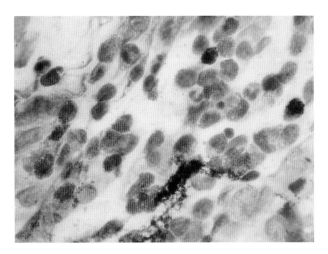

Figura 7.61 Allergic rhinitis. Immuno-inflammatory infiltrate (MGG staining; ×1000).

in allergic patients is a sign of bacterial superinfection (**Fig. 7.63**).

Treatment Strategies in Allergic Rhinitis

Nasal cytology should be regarded as more than a simple diagnostic study because it can also be employed to monitor medical treatment of nasal diseases. In the past decade, the literature has emphasized this aspect, describing the reduction in immuno-inflammatory cells and bacteria, as well as degranulation processes owing to treatment strategies using drugs including: corticosteroids, local and systemic antihistamines, chromoglycates, antibiotics, vasoconstrictors and so forth.

The routine use of cytologic determination is broadly supported by it being inexpensive and non invasive.

In allergic rhinitis, citology is particularly important in treatment planning with its ability to detect a disease in the preclinical stage and to follow its course through to the post-clinical stage. In both these stages, history taking and physical examination are unremarkable, even though immuno-inflammatory processes associated with cytologic alterations are present in the mucosa. This residual *inflammation*, if persistent (and also sometimes complicated by bacterial superinfection), has a poor prognosis, indicating that the disease will progress toward a chronic course or additional complications (**Fig. 7.64**).

Acute clinical manifestations call for prompt medical treatment, which can sometimes be aggressive or inappropriate (e.g. *overtreatment*), to manage abnormal clinical events and pathogenic pro-

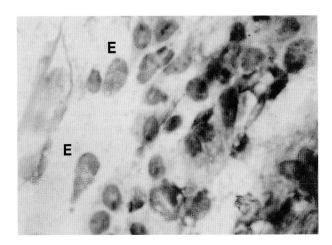

Figure 7.62 Allergic rhinitis. Immuno-inflammatory infiltrate with prominent eosinophils (E) (MGG staining; ×1000).

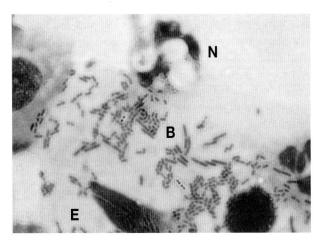

Figure 7.63 Allergic rhinitis. Bacterial superinfection. Bacterial colony (B), neutrophil (N), eosinophil (E) (MGG staining; ×1000 with CMF 2.2×).

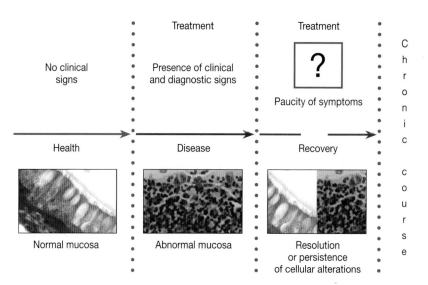

Figure 7.64 Correlation between clinical and cytologic findings.

cesses, while minimal persistent inflammation often eludes therapy.

The consequence is that it can continue to initiate or exacerbate tissue damage through the continued release of proinflammatory cytokines, leading to recurrent activation of immuno-inflammatory cells and their prolonged survival in a self-perpetuating cycle of stimulus and response.

On the basis of cytologic evidence diagnostic for a certain disorder (e.g. allergic rhinitis), a treatment strategy can be appropriately formulated and response to therapy monitored during the course of the disease, particularly when persistent inflammation is latent and asymptomatic.

It is important to consider that prophylactic treatment of pollinosis (hayfever), when guided by the nasal cytogram, will ensure the two advantages of a more positive clinical course of the disease and reduced treatment duration, thereby improving the patient's quality of life. This also reduces healthcare costs by preventing the condition from becoming chronic and accompanying comorbidities and avoiding.

In asymptomatic stages, treatment planning is difficult because nasal allergies are seldom diagnosed by conventional clinical and diagnostic procedures. The only effective means of detecting latent disease is, in fact, by cytologic study of the nasal mucosa, which can reveal the cells involved in certain pathogenic processes.

Despite the absence of clinical symptoms in such circumstances, it is important to realize that we are nevertheless confronted by an active disease requiring prompt medical treatment (**Fig. 7.65**).

On the other hand no treatment is necessary when clinical signs and symptoms are absent and the nasal cytogram is negative. In seasonal allergic rhinitis, preventive therapy is with disodium cromoglycate (DSCG). It is widely recognized that this agent has therapeutic efficacy only when administered in the prepollen phase, i.e. before cytologic and clinical signs of inflammation develop. Since DSCG has a stabilizing effect on the cell membrane, administration is recommended at least 50-60 days before the estimated start of the pollen season based on the pollen calendar of previous seasons. In all forms of the hayfever, this treatment induces a more favorable clinical course (improved relief of symptoms and shorter duration of therapy) in acute phase rhinitis.

In patients without symptoms or with mild to moderate symptoms accompanied by sporadic eosinophils but with degranulation, local corticosteroids are recommended (budesonide, fluticasone furoate, momethasone furoate, etc.) along with local (azelastine) or systemic antihistamines (cetirizine, desloatadine, ebastine, loratadine, levocetirizine, rupatadine, etc.). Only elevated eosinophil and mast cell levels accompanied by degranulation and severe clinical symptoms (serious nasal congestion, rhinorrhea, sneezing and general malaise) warrant the use of systemic corticosteroids (deflazacort, prednisone, etc.), which should be continued until symptoms resolve and the nasal cytogram indicates partial or complete remission of the acute state. Therapy is then continued with topical corticosteroids and systemic antihistamines for at least 30 days to manage the minimal residual inflammation that follows a major allergy attack.

Finally, specific immunotherapy (SIT) represents the true causal treatment of allergic rhinitis.

SIT is indicated in pollen-induced respiratory al-

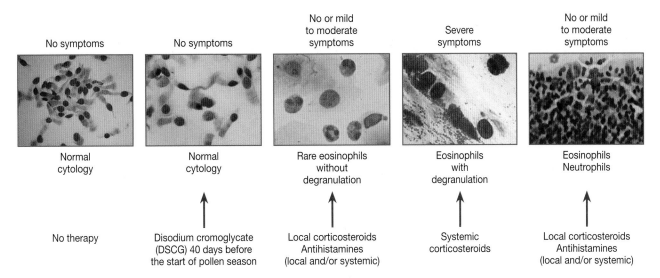

No symptoms	No symptoms	No or mild to moderate symptoms	Severe symptoms	No or mild to moderate symptoms
Normal cytology	Normal cytology	Rare eosinophils without degranulation	Eosinophils with degranulation	Eosinophils Neutrophils
No therapy	Disodium cromoglycate (DSCG) 40 days before the start of pollen season	Local corticosteroids Antihistamines (local and/or systemic)	Systemic corticosteroids	Local corticosteroids Antihistamines (local and/or systemic)

Figure 7.65 Cytologic evaluation aimed at instituting a more rational treatment strategy in allergic rhinitis.

lergies depending on the severity of the symptoms and the duration of the exposure. In the case of short season allergies, such as cypress or olive pollen allergies, providing the prescription of SIT is strongly supported by its cost-benefit ratio, it is preferable to perform vaccination before the pollen season starts, beginning three months beforehand. SIT is also indicated when the underlying disease is associated with asthma and oculorhinitis.

Particular consideration should be given to patients suffering from "overlapping" rhinopathies (e.g. NARES + cypress pollen-induced allergic rhinitis) – this topic will be addressed later –, who are clearly not ideal candidates for SIT. Patients with a "dual" pathology, if submitted to SIT, will show only limited symptom improvements, because of the overlapping non allergic disease. The specialist's role, therefore, is to clarify the prognosis, i.e. real clinical benefits that such treatment can be expected to bring over the years.

Non Allergic ("Cellular") Vasomotor Rhinitis

In the setting of chronic rhinopathies, the category of non allergic ("cellular") rhinitis continues to be unclear and lacking an unambiguous clinical-diagnostic and therapeutic approach. These variants are often not diagnosed and, as a result, are labeled "non specific" vasomotor rhinitis. With the exception of the neutrophilic forms, they are "congenital" diseases and thus present at birth. Failure to identify them is linked solely to the fact that nasal cytology is not included among the routine battery of neonatal investigations! They account for around 15% of all nasal diseases, which is quite a considerable proportion, and are usually accompanied by intense pseudo-allergic symptoms (nasal congestion, itching, bouts of sneezing, a sensation of burning of the nasal mucosa, rhinorrhea, etc.), that often leads them to be confused with IgE-mediated rhinitis. Patients also present a non-specific reactivity that manifests itself with the onset of symptoms in the presence of various stimuli (changes of temperature, cold air, strong smells, cigarette smoke, nasal irrigation, topical drug treatments, etc.). Also they are often forced to give up sporting pursuits on account of the onset of intense nasal hyperreactivity (sneezing, nasal congestion and burning) when the nasal mucosa comes into contact with certain substances (chlorinated swimming pool water). In addition they complain of nasal congestion, often a bascula, which is accentuated during sleep, causing snoring and oral breathing, and hyperreactivity of the nasal mucosa, evoked mainly by non specific stimuli. When obtaining the history of patients with these forms of rhinitis it is typical to find that they have undergone many specialty consultations (ENT specialists, allergists, pediatricians, pulmonologists) before finally obtaining the definitive diagnosis. Nasal obturation may be in fact, this anamnestic aspect might even be considered "pathognomonic" of these forms of rhinitis. They are not likely to be diagnosed with a first ENT consultation especially when comprhensive investigatory tools are not employed i.e. accurate rhinologic and allergologic diagnosis (history taking, skin prick test, nasal endoscopy, nasal cytology, rhinomanometry, specific nasal provocation test, etc., **Fig. 7.66**). Given that these are diseases with a "cellular" expression, the diagnostic gold standard is clearly cytology of the nasal mucosa.

These patients will frequently have a family history of asthma and/or nasal polyposis and a past history of surgery on the turbinates, aimed at solving the "blocked nose" symptom. These interventions very often prove to be ineffective and even harmful, resulting in scarring (formation of synechiae between the turbinate and the septum), crusting rhinitis, and mucosal atrophy (even leading to empty nose syndrome). This is because they do not target the etiopathogenetic cause: infiltration of eosinophils and/or mast cells. Another typical feature of these conditions is excessive use of nasal decongestants, trying to resolve the chronic nasal congestion. It must be remembered that the chronic use of these drugs may lead to the development of rhinitis medicamentosa, which will overlap the pre-existing rhinitis.

These conditions, because of their intense and persistent nasal symptoms, and tendency to co-occur with other symptoms and with important systemic diseases (bronchial asthma, sensitivity to acetylsalicylic acid, rhinobronchial syndrome, nasal polyposis, rhinosinusitis). These are associated with significant detrimental effects on quality of life, increased costs (specialist medical examinations, laboratory and instrumental examinations, drugs not reimbursed by the national health system, etc.).

Finally, since these entities constitute *chronic* diseases, they require chronic treatments and personalized follow-up programs, aimed at controlling the symptoms and preventing complications (rhinosinusitis, polyposis, asthma, etc.). Therefore, it is important to give the patient clear and comprehensive information on the disease and the therapeutic program, clarifying the strengths and limitations of these drug treatments in terms of control of the disease; this is to ensure maximum adherence to the assigned treatment program, and avoid raising false hopes of a definitive cure.

The "cellular" forms of rhinitis are divided, according to their cytotype, into non allergic rhinitis with neutrophils (NARNE), non allergic rhinitis with eosinophilia syndrome (NARES), non allergic rhinitis with mast cells (NARMA), and non allergic rhinitis with eosinophils and mast cells (NARESMA) (**Fig. 7.67**).

Non Allergic Rhinitis with Neutrophils (NARNE)

NARNE is characterized microscopically by major infiltration of neutrophils (> 30%). Unlike what is observed in infectious rhinitis, the neutrophils are

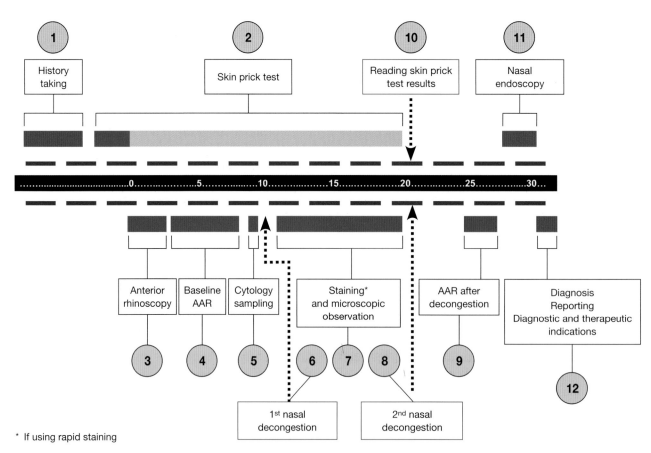

* If using rapid staining

Figure 7.66 Sequence of the rhinologic and allergy diagnostic work up (AAR, active anterior rhinomanometry).

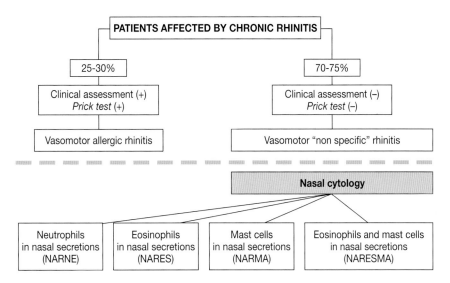

Figure 7.67 In the diagnostic algorithm for rhinitis, nasal cytology makes it possible to diagnose special nosologic entities that are otherwise labeled "non-specific".

not accompanied by the presence of bacteria, spores and fungal hyphae (**Fig. 7.68 a-b**).

The increased incidence of this rhinopathy, especially in recent years, is probably linked to physical and chemical insult to of the mucosa, since the subjects most affected seem to be industrial and craft workers, people living in industrialized areas, and chronic smokers.

It is often found in patients with gastroesophageal reflux disease, wherein the exhalation of hydrochloric acid and its subsequent contact with the nasal mucosa explains the recruitment of these inflammatory cells. The prolonged presence and continuous release of chemical mediators (in particular neutrophil elastase) are the main cause of free radical formation and consequent impairment of the mucosal epithelium, which is translated clinically into "vaso-

motor" symptoms (seromucous rhinorrhea, sneezing bouts, burning sensation and nasal congestion).

Unlike the other "cellular" vasomotor forms (NARMA, NARES and NARESMA), the symptoms are far less intense and can regress once the pathogenic cause has been identified and removed.

Non Allergic Rhinitis with Eosinophilia Syndrome (NARES)

NARES is a non IgE-mediated vasomotor rhinitis, characterized by eosinophilic infiltration of the nasal mucosa, which usually reaches relatively high proportions (50-70%) (**Fig. 7.69**).

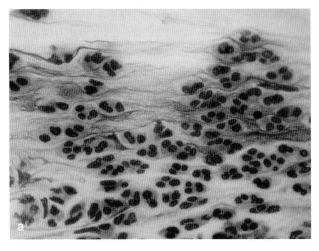
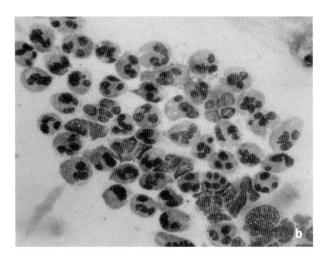

Figure 7.68 a-b Non allergic rhinitis with neutrophils (NARNE). The rhinocytogram is characterized by numerous neutrophils (MGG staining; ×1000).

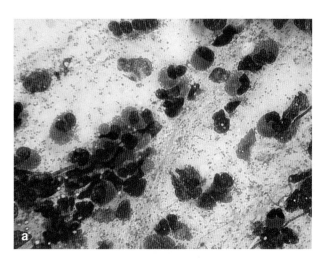
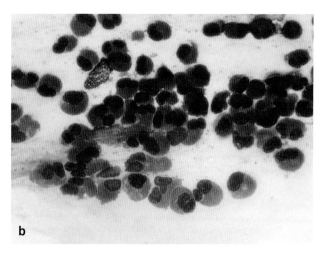

Figure 7.69 a-b Eosinophilic infiltration of the nasal mucosa (NARES) (MGG staining; ×1000).

Like NARMA and NARESMA it often co-occurs with nasal polyposis, and/or asthma, and/or sensitivity to acetylsalicylic acid.

In a proportion of patients, the nasal eosinophilia is accompanied by blood hypereosinophilia.

Sometimes, these forms of rhinopathy can recruit, for reasons that are still unknown, mast cells, thereby turning into eosinophilic-mast cell forms (NARESMA), in which the symptoms become more intense and continuous.

Non Allergic Rhinitis with Mast Cells (NARMA)

Microscopically, this rhinopathy is characterized by the presence of mast cells in the nasal mucosa, partially degranulated (**Fig. 7.70**). The clinical pre-

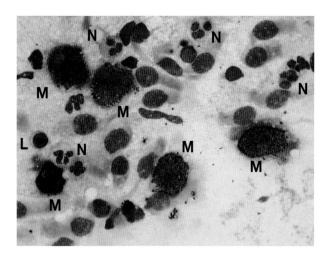

Figure 7.70 Non allergic rhinitis with mast cells (NARMA). The microscopic picture is dominated by numerous mast cells (M). In the field of view there are also a few neutrophils (N) and occasional lymphocyte (L) (MGG staining; ×1000).

sentation is very intense (nasal congestion, rhinorrhea, sneezing bouts, nasal itching) and it is often associated with the presence of asthma and/or nasal-sinus polyposis.

Like NARES, NARMA can be a transitional form leading to NARESMA.

Non Allergic Rhinitis with Eosinophils and Mast Cells (NARESMA)

NARESMA is a disease entity that has only recently been identified and described, which, like NARES, NARMA and NARNE, is part of the "cellular" group of nasal diseases. Cytologically it is characterized by the presence of eosinophils and mast cells, in varying proportions, and marked degranulation (**Fig. 7.71**).

The most important aspect of NARESMA is that, unlike the other forms described above, it is more frequently associated with nasal polyposis, asthma, rhinosinusitis, etc., as well as with a more impaired quality of life, partly due to sleep disorders (frequent awakenings, snoring and sleep apnea). If associated with nasal polyposis, it represents a less favorable progress for relapse.

NARESMA, like NARES and NARMA, responds well to corticosteroid therapy, both topical and systemic and, like all the forms of vasomotor rhinitis, it requires frequent clinical-cytologic monitoring.

"Overlapping" Rhinopathies

In the field of nasal diagnostics, the most important contribution made by nasal cytology in recent years has been, in my view, the introduction of the new concept of "overlapping" rhinopathies. Indeed, thanks to diagnostic cytology it is now possible to identify patients who are affected by more than one diagnostic entity (e.g., by allergic rhinitis associated with NARES, or allergic rhinitis associated with NARESMA, etc.). From a clinical point of view, these patients, despite testing positive for one or more "seasonal" allergens, have "persistent" nasal symptoms, together with a rhinocytogram showing the presence of eosinophils and/or mast cells, even outside the pollen season. In these cases, nasal cytology is extremely useful, as it is the only diagnostic study capable of "unmasking" these clinical conditions.

Diagnosis of these forms of rhinitis is crucially important, especially in the field of Allergy, where therapeutic strategies range from pharmacologic approaches (antihistamines, corticosteroids, leukotriene modifiers, decongestants, etc) to specific immunotherapy (SIT), not to mention prevention, where every therapeutic response should be interpreted with extreme caution.

In this regard, it is worth remembering that though most patients with overlapping rhinopathies treated by SIT alone will obtain all the benefits associated with this treatment (arrest of the "allergic march" and of the evolution toward polysensitization), they will not experience, at the end of the 3-5 years of therapy, significant improvements in their symptoms. This is because SIT has no effect on the concomitant "non IgE-mediated" rhinopathy. In these cases, it will always be necessary to combine the SIT with a pharmacologic therapy (topical and/or systemic corticosteroids and, in some cases, leukotriene modifiers) in order to control the symptoms.

Therefore, a thorough rhinologic and allergologic diagnostic work up (**Fig. 7.72**), also designed to identify the presence of clinical and cytologic signs that might raise suspicion of "overlapping" rhinopathies (**Tab. 7.4**), will allow the specialist to make an accurate diagnosis, which is essential in order to plan a targeted therapeutic strategy. Furthermore, before prescribing a treatment program, which in these cases will always be long term, the patient must be given clear and exhaustive information on his "particular" condition. All this may help to avoid false hopes of a definitive cure, and encourage greater compliance with the treatment and with the schedule of outpatient checks.

Nasal Cytology in the Diagnostic Strategy of Vasomotor Rhinitis

Cytologic study is an essential diagnostic aid to differentiate between numerous rhinopathies, and

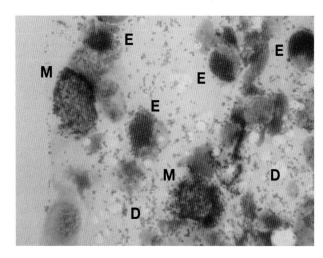

Figure 7.71 Non allergic rhinitis with eosinophils and mast cells (NARESMA). The microscopic picture is dominated by numerous eosinophils (E), mast cells (M) and marked degranulation (D) (MGG staining; ×1000 with CMF 1.4×).

to facilitate their recognition in conditions where neither symptoms nor allergy testing prove capable of discerning the diagnosis of a certain nasal disease.

In addition to evaluation of symptoms and clinical assessment, history taking remains a key tool in the diagnosis of nasal diseases, with attention directed at discovering a positive family history of atopic disorders. Within this context, cytologic study can reveal cell changes suggestive of nasal diseases.

A diagnostic algorithm making it possible to initiate a strategic approach to treating nasal diseases is illustrated in **figure 7.72**.

In perennial allergic rhinitis, the nasal cytogram demonstrates a predominance of neutrophils followed, in decreasing order, by eosinophils, lymphocytes and rare mast cells.

This reflects a condition of *minimal persistent inflammation* usually accompanied by mild clinical symptoms, chiefly in the form of nasal congestion and rhinorrhea.

Degranulation is difficult to detect microscopically, except during periods of peak allergen levels when clinical symptoms become more pronounced with the development of itching and sneezing.

Whenever the skin prick test is positive and the nasal cytogram is negative, even in peak pollen periods, the diagnosis is *ASA-"sensitive" vasomotor rhinitis*. This disorder requires close clinical monitoring and regular cytology determinations (every 6 to 12 months) to promptly detect the transformation from ASA-sensitivity into an allergic condition.

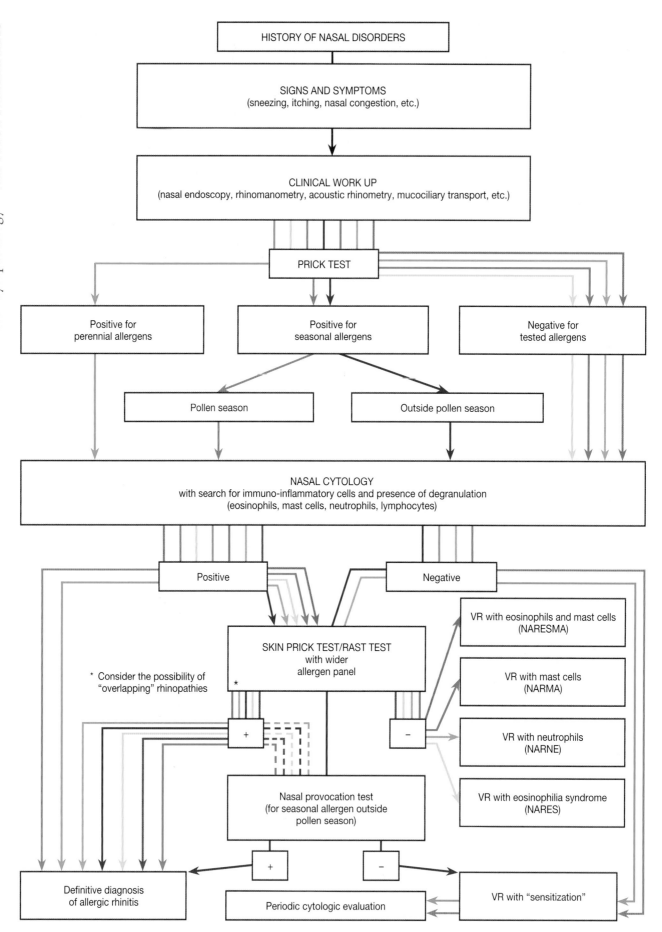

Figure 7.72 Diagnostic algorithm for vasomotor rhinitis (VR).

Table 7.4 When to suspect "overlapping" of different rhinopathies (allergic rhinitis + NARESMA, NARES or NARMA)

Clinical criteria

- Chronic "vasomotor" rhinitis symptoms (nasal congestion, rhinorrhea, sneezing a salve), present even outside the pollen season, in a patient with positive skin prick test and/or RAST test

- Increased "vasomotor"-type nasal reactivity to non specific stimuli (sudden changes in temperature, light stimuli, strong smells, cigarette smoke, exposure to chlorine (swimming), etc.)

- Disturbances of taste and smell (suspect onset of nasal polyposis)

- Positive family history of nasal polyposis, NARES, NARMA, NARESMA, asthma, sensitivity to acetylsalicylic acid, hypo-anosmia, vasomotor rhinitis labeled "non specific", previous turbinate surgery for nasal congestion which gave poor medium- to long-term results

- Recurrent use of nasal decongestants

- Little or no clinical benefit following turbinate surgery for nasal congestion

- Little or no clinical benefit following a cycle of specific immunotherapy (SIT)

Cytologic criteria

- In the *forms with "persistent" symptoms*, overlapping should be suspected in all patients with a rhinocytogram showing a cell profile different from that associated with "persistent minimal inflammation" (i.e. different from that characterised by numerous neutrophils, some lymphocytes and occasional eosinophils, with rare signs of degranulation), where there are eosinophils > 20% and/or mast cells > 10%.

- In the *forms with "intermittent" symptoms*, overlapping should be suspected in all patients with a positive rhinocytogram (eosinophils > 20% and/or mast cells > 10%) outside the pollen season for the allergen/s identified by allergy testing (skin prick test and/or RAST test).

In rhinocytology, November tends to be preferred for "unraveling" overlapping rhinopathies, as this is the month in which most airborne pollens are absent.
The presence of immuno-inflammatory cells (eosinophils and/or mast cells) associated with rhinitis symptoms confirms the presence of overlapping diseases.

RAST, *radio-allergo-sorbent test*.

Another important point to consider in seasonal allergic rhinitis is that diagnostic evaluation may be performed in two different periods of the year: during and outside the pollen season. In the former, a patient with allergic rhinitis presents with all the clinical signs of the disorder. The nasal cytogram shows a prevalence of eosinophils, with mast cells in partial or complete degranulation, as typically occurs in pollen-induced forms, as well as the presence of numerous neutrophils. But when the patient is evaluated outside the pollen season, the clinical and cytologic conditions are silent, especially if the pollen season ended at least 60 days prior to the examination. To establish a clear diagnosis in such cases, a nasal provocation test (Allerkin®) should be performed using the suspected allergen.

Particular attention should also be paid to patients with a positive skin prick test for seasonal allergens and a positive nasal cytogram for immuno-inflammatory cells even outside the pollen season (in such cases it is necessary to consider a form in which there is an overlapping of two diseases: allergic rhinitis + "cellular" non allergic rhinitis), as well as those with negative skin prick test and positive nasal cytogram. In both situations, the skin prick test should be repeated with a wider allergen panel in order to identify the allergen responsible for the mucosal cell excitation.

A positive skin prick test should be followed by confirmation of the diagnosis using nasal provocation tests with the suspected allergen, performed outside the pollen season and delivered to mucosa not showing immuno-inflammatory cells.

In addition to providing a definitive diagnosis of allergic rhinitis, nasal cytology can help identify other clinically relevant conditions. All nasal diseases in which the skin prick test is negative (whether using a basic or an expanded allergen panel), but the nasal cytogram is positive for immuno-inflammatory cells, can be classified according to the predominance of the cell type as: *Non Allergic Vasomotor Rhinitis with Neutrophils* (NARNE), *Non-Specific Vasomotor Rhinitis with Eosinophilia Syndrome* (NARES), *Non-Specific Vasomotor Rhinitis with Mast Cells* (NARMA) or *Non Allergic Vasomotor Rhinitis with Eosinophils and Mast Cells* (NARESMA) (**Fig. 7.72**).

We end this chapter with **table 7.5**, which shows the cytologic findings in the different rhinopaties.

Table 7.5   Nasal cytology in various clinical conditions

	Eosinophils	Mast cells	Neutrophils	Bacteria	Fungal spores	Infectious spot	Ciliated cells
Normal	0	0	0 – 1+	0	0	0	N SHS+
Allergic rhinitis	1 – 4+	1 – 4+	1 – 4+	0	0	0	Decreased SHS–
NARES	1 – 4+	0	PP	0	0	0	Decreased SHS–
NARESMA	1 – 4+	1 – 4+	PP	0	0	0	Decreased SHS–
Mast cell rhinitis	0	1 – 4+	PP	0	0	0	Decreased SHS–
Irritant rhinitis (neutrophil)	0	0	1 – 4+	0	0	0	Decreased SHS–
Rhinosinusitis	0	0	1 – 4+	1 – 4+	0	Present	Decreased SHS–
Viral rhinitis	0	0	1 – 4+	0	0	0	CCP - MNC
Fungal rhinitis	0	0	1 – 4+	0	1 – 4+	Present	Decreased SHS–
Nasal polyposis	1 – 4+	0 – 4+	PP	PP	PP	PP	Decreased SHS–
Antrochoanal polyp	0	0	1 – 4+	PP	PP	PP	Decreased SHS–
Rhinitis medicamentosa	0	0	0 – 1+	0	0	0	N SHS+
Pregnancy rhinitis	0	0	0 – 1+	0	0	0	N SHS+
Atrophic rhinitis	0	0	1 – 4+	0	0	0	Squamous metaplasia

N, denotes normal; PP, possible presence; SHS, supranuclear hyperchromatic stria; CCP, ciliocytophthoria; MNC, multinucleation; original data from Meltzer EO, et al., 1999 (adapted).

HYPERPLASTIC/GRANULOMATOUS RHINITIS

Nasal-Sinus Polyposis

Nasal polyps are protuberances of the mucosa that appear pale, translucent, gelatinous, smooth, and round or pyriform. They occur most frequently in the middle meatus and in the anterior ethmoid region. Histology reveals an edematous structure containing scattered masses of lymphocytes, plasma cells, eosinophils and mast cells, covered with a ciliated-type pseudostratified epithelium. To a greater or lesser extent these alterations also involve the surrounding mucosa of the nasal and paranasal sinuses, as demonstrated by computed tomography and magnetic resonance imaging. A typical feature is the involvement of the mucosa of the ethmoid and maxillary sinuses, with thickening or polypoid degeneration. Recent studies have clarified, definitively and unequivocally, that nasal polyposis is not related to atopy, or to any complication of atopy. This is confirmed by the fact that the rate of allergic rhinitis in polyposis is around 30%, which is comparable to epidemiological data collected in the general population. The prevalence of nasal polyposis is about 30% in patients with bronchial asthma and 50% in those with ASA-sensitive asthma. The mean age at diagnosis is 30-50 years. The pathogenetic mechanism is unknown.

It is our belief that nasal polyposis constitutes a hyperplastic-degenerative espression of the nasal mucosa, secondary to a chronic "cellular" rhinopathy (NARES, NARMA, NARESMA) that (since these conditions are hardly ever diagnosed) has gone un-

treated. Only longitudinal studies will confirm this etiopathogenetic hypothesis.

It is however supported by the fact that the nasal cytology is characterized by a predominance of intact or degranulated eosinophils (**Fig. 7.73**), mast cells (**Fig. 7.74**) and, in a high percentage of cases, by both cytotypes showing partial or total degranulation.

It is rare to find a "neutrophilic"cytology (**Fig. 7.75**), as is typically present in polyposis of patients with cystic fibrosis, in antrochoanal polyps and in inverted papilloma (in these latter two forms almost always unilaterally).

Nasal congestion accompanying nasal polyps is a

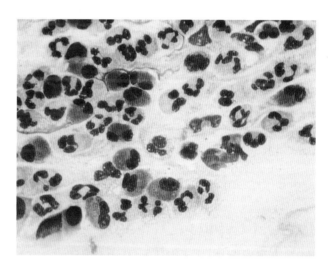

Figure 7.73 Nasal polyposis. Polyp with numerous eosinophils in nasal discharge. The skin prick test was negative (MGG staining; ×1000).

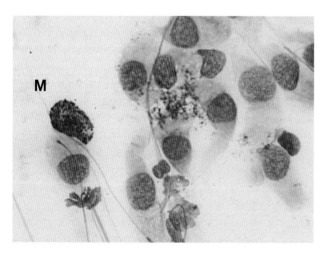

Figure 7.74 Nasal polyposis. Nasal polyposis in a patient with nasal mastocytosis and negative skin prick test. Mast cell (M) (MGG staining; ×1000).

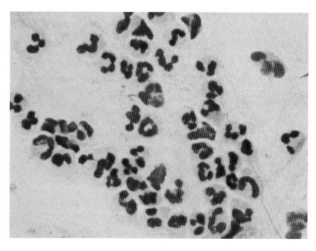

Figure 7.75 Antrochoanal polyp. Specimen characterized by neutrophilia (MGG staining; ×1000).

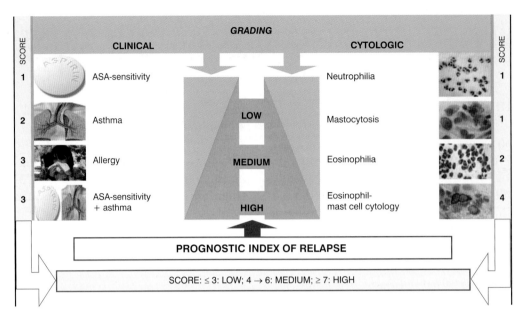

Figure 7.76   Nasal-sinus polyposis: from clinical-cytologic grading to prognostic index of relapse.

predisposing factor for the development of infection and sinusitis; therefore, bacterial colonies on the cytologic smear will confirm suspected infection and should prompt appropriate medical treatment. Treatment is repeated nasal lavage with saline solution warmed to body temperature and performed using an irrigation system such as NAS-IR® for effective cleaning of the mucosa. This is an essential first step prior to administration of a topical agent (corticosteroids, antibiotics, decongestants, antihistamines, etc.).

Clinical-Cytologic Grading and Prognostic Index of Relapse

Despite advances in microendoscopic surgical treatment, the problem of post-surgical relapse of nasal-sinus polyposis, which occurs in 23% to 87% of cases, remains unresolved. However, the risk of recurrence does not seem to be linked to the type of intervention, but rather depends on factors that are only partially known.

A number of studies have attempted to identify "negative" prognostic factors as the causes of post-surgical relapse of nasal polyposis. Some of these were not significant (age, gender, septal deviations, atopic status, type of surgery). Others have been found by some investigators, but not all, to be significant (asthma, intolerance of aspirin [ASA-sensitivity] and of NSAIDs, extent of polyposis, percentage of eosinophils in the chorion, previous nasal polypectomy, Widal's syndrome, the presence of mast cells in polyps, and increased IgE levels associated with increased eosinophils).

In light of this, we recently conducted a study seeking to expand this research through investigations both at the cellular level, using the technique of nasal mucosal scraping, and at the clinical level (ASA-sensitivity, asthma, allergy, ASA-sensitivity + asthma).

Our results are in agreement with the literature, the correlation between ASA-sensitivity/number of nasal polypectomies was not found to be significant. Similar results were obtained for the correlations between Widal's syndrome and number of polypectomies, and the correlation between asthma alone and number of polypectomies.

Conversely, significant correlations did emerge when comparing some clinical parameters (allergy, asthma, ASA-sensitivity, ASA-sensitivity + asthma) with cytologic findings (neutrophilia, eosinophilia, mastocytosis, eosinophil-mast cell cytology). From this analysis it was possible to obtain a clinical-cytologic grading (CCG) system, whose final score expresses the prognostic index of relapse (PIR), which, in different cases, may be low, medium or high (**Fig. 7.76**).

In light of these studies, it is desirable that all patients affected by nasal-sinus polyps be classified, following a full preoperative clinical-cytologic assessment, according to their CCG score and relative PIR. This would make it possible to achieve two objectives:
- it would "steer" the otorhinolaryngologist toward a more rational approach to the medical-surgical treatment and subsequent follow up of these patients;
- it would allow the patient to gain a better understanding of his disease and its evolutionary aspects, avoiding false hopes of a definitive cure and encouraging greater compliance with the personalized medical treatment and with the schedule of outpatient checks, which are crucial in order to control the disease and prevent complications.

OTHER RHINITIS

Pregnancy Rhinitis

Suspected causes of pregnancy rhinitis are estrogens and progesterones that stimulate glandular hypersecretion and increase blood volume in the nasal tissues resulting in mucosal hypertrophy which causes higher nasal resistance.

Rhinitis Medicamentosa

Rhinitis medicamentosa is chiefly caused by the chronic use of nasal vasoconstrictors.

It is worth pointing out that rhinitis medicamentosa does not just happens. If a patient is repeatedly using a nasal decongestant, this is usually because there is an underlying nasal disease, yet to be diagnosed.

It is worth noting that in both these forms of vasomotor rhinitis no alterations in cellular components are found, unless associated with coexisting disorders (allergy or infection).

Atrophic Rhinitis

Atrophic rhinitis is a chronic nasal disorder characterized by atrophy of the mucosal and submucosal epithelia. Causal agents were once thought to be *Perez's Coccobacillus* and *Klebsiella ozaenae* but these are now considered secondary organisms.

Atrophic rhinitis occurs less frequently than in the past, perhaps owing to improved living and sanitary conditions; however, in areas of Eastern Europe and India it is still endemic.

Since it has a predilection for young women, some investigators have suspected hormonal factors, while others claim the condition arises from auto-immune mechanisms triggered by a virus, impaired defense or vitamin deficiency.

On physical examination, the turbinates appear atrophied and the nasal cavities abnormally wide. Abundant exudate forms crusts covering part of the nasal mucosa, and crust-free areas appear dry and opaque. In the *senile chronic rhinopathy* variant, transformation of the epithelial mucosa tends toward replacement of normal differentiated cells with squamous cells (*atrophic transformation*) (**Fig. 7.77**).

In patients with atrophic rhinitis, the cytogram is characterized by various degrees of epithelial squamous metaplasia and chronic infiltration by inflammatory cells.

Diffuse squamous metaplasia is accompanied by a reduction in seromucosal glands and goblet cells.

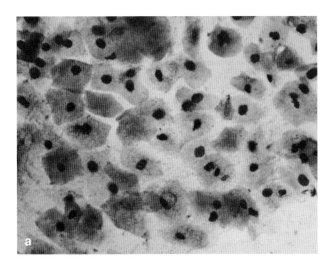 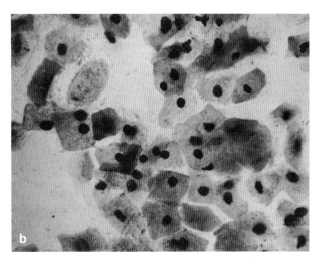

Figure 7.77 a-b Squamous metaplasia in a patient with atrophic rhinitis (MGG staining; ×1000).

CONCLUSION

The importance of and interest in nasal cytology as a diagnostic tool in nasal disease have greatly increased. Modern methods of sample collection, staining and interpretation have been standardized. These have contributed to our ability to differentiate chronic nasal diseases, monitor their course and plan more rational ways to treat them.

I hope that this clinical atlas will encourage wider interest in nasal cytology, a technique that has been recognized for over a century as a valid diagnostic procedure that can provide an important link between cell pathophysiology and the clinical field.

I wish to acknowledge the work of pioneers in nasal cytology such as Bizzozero, Eyrmann, Gollash and Bryan, along with that of contemporary researchers such as Anderson, Bickmore, Ciprandi, Cohen, Connell, Durham, Hansel, Jacobs, Jalowayski, Lans, Meltzer, Mygind, Naclerio, Orgel, Pipkorn, Settipane, Zeiger and the many others who have significantly contributed to advancing scientific research and clinical applications of nasal cytology.

Photomicrographic Images of Normal and Abnormal Nasal Cytology

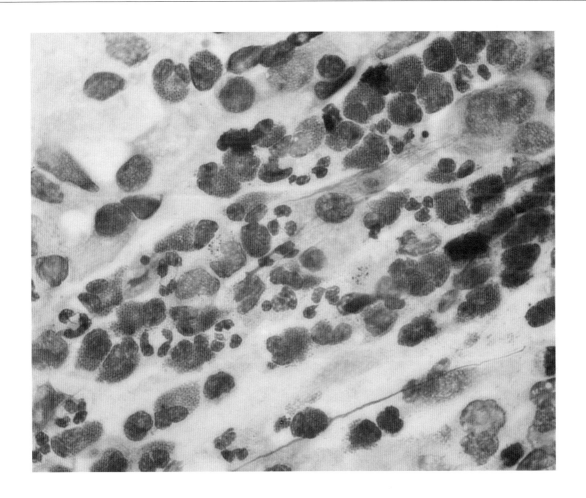

Longitudinal studies in nasal cytology
may confirm, in not many years from now, the etiopathogenetic hypothesis
that is present in the following expression:

"I was born with NARES... twenty years later
I was diagnosed with nasal polyps"

Matteo Gelardi, 2010

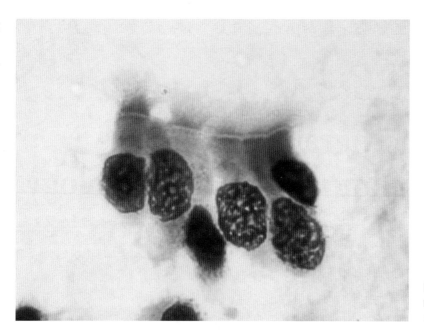

Figure 8.1 Group of ciliated cells with nuclei at various heights (MGG staining; ×1000 with CMF 1×).

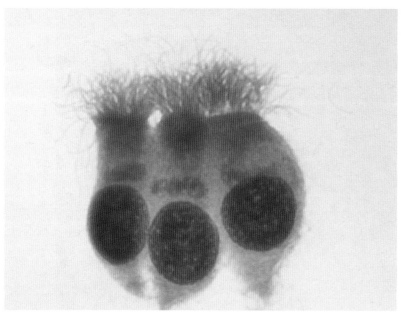

Figure 8.2 Ciliated cells with prominent ciliary apparatus. The supranuclear hyperchromatic stria is clearly visible (SHS+) (MGG staining; ×1000 with CMF 2×).

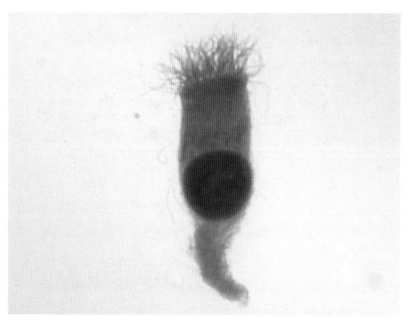

Figure 8.3 Ciliated cell. Ciliary apparatus and basal portion are well preserved (MGG staining; ×1000 with CMF 2×).

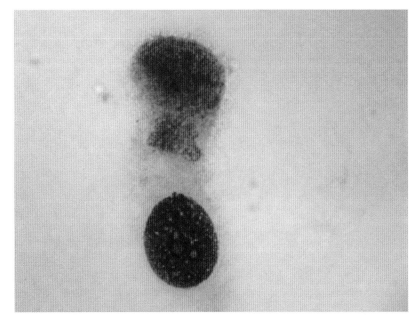

Figure 8.4 Columnar cells of the nasal mucosa. The two nucleoli inside the nucleus can clearly be seen (MGG staining; ×1000 with CMF 2×).

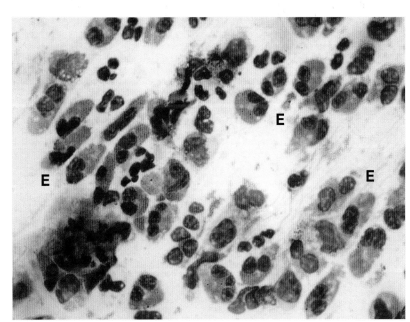

Figure 8.5 Allergic rhinitis in acute phase: numerous eosinophils (E), partly degranulated (MGG staining; ×1000).

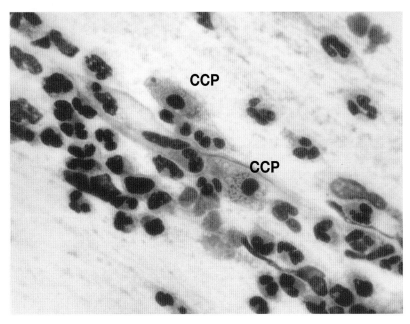

Figure 8.6 Viral rhinits: columnar cells with signs of ciliocytophthoria (CCP, ciliocytophthoria) (MGG staining; ×1000).

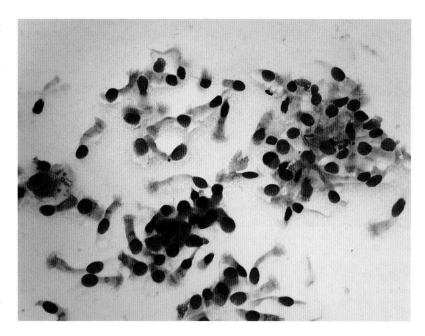

Figure 8.7 Normal cytology. Numerous ciliated cells with prominent ciliary apparatus (MGG staining; ×400).

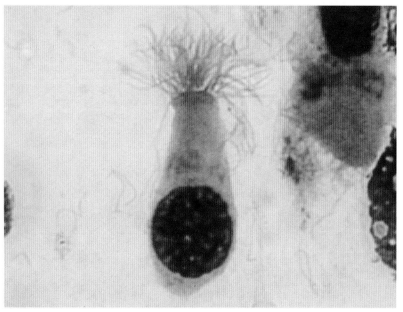

Figure 8.8 Ciliated cell with prominent ciliary apparatus and reduction of supranuclear hyperchromatic stria (SHS) (MGG staining; ×1000 with CMF 2×).

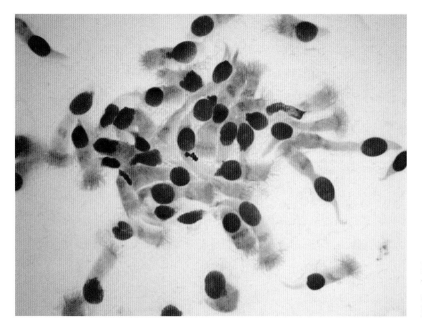

Figure 8.9 Normal cytology. Ciliated cell with prominent ciliary apparatus (same cytological smear as in Figure 8.7 at higher magnification; MGG staining).

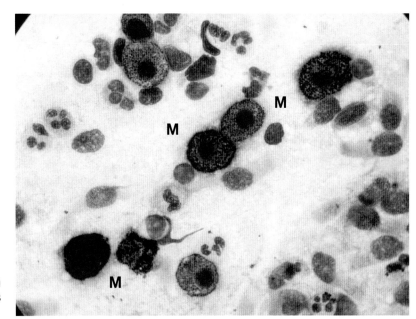

Figure 8.10 Non allergic rhinitis with mast cells (NARMA): numerous mast cells (M) (MGG staining; ×1000).

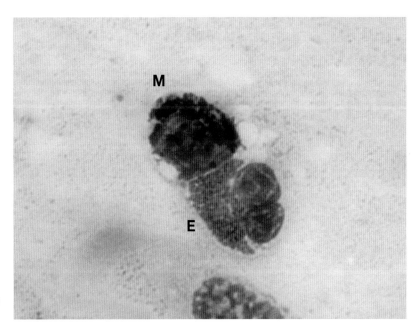

Figure 8.11 Mast cell (M), eosinophil (E) (MGG staining; ×1000 with CMF 2.2×).

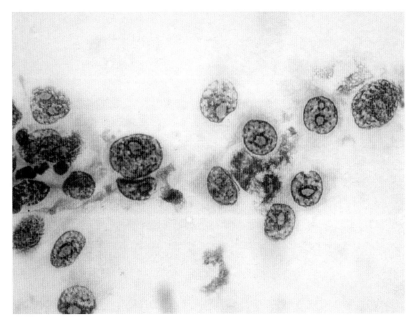

Figure 8.12 Metaplastic cells: it is easy to identify the nuclei and the nucleoli they contain (light blue) (MGG staining; ×1000).

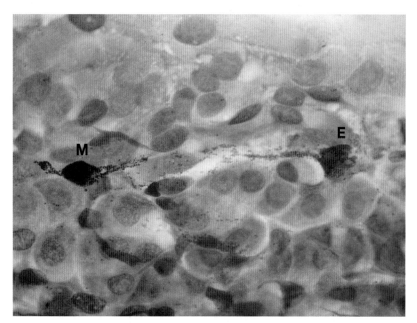

Figure 8.13 Allergic rhinitis. Eosinophil (E) and degranulating mast cell (M), surrounded by numerous metaplastic cells (MGG staining; ×1000).

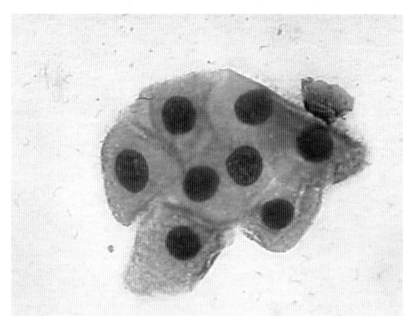

Figure 8.14 Squamous cell (MGG staining; ×1000 with CMF 1.4×).

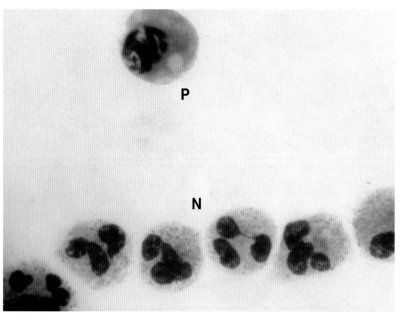

Figure 8.15 Several neutrophils (N) and a plasma cell (P) (MGG staining; ×1000 with CMF 2×).

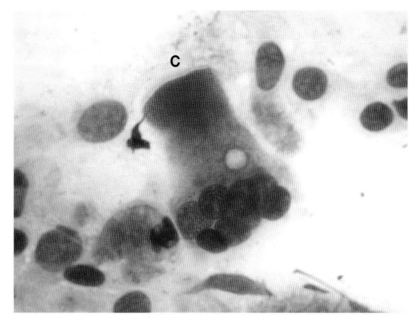

Figure 8.16 Viral rhinitis. Polynucleated columnar cell (C) (MGG staining; ×1000 with CMF 1.2×).

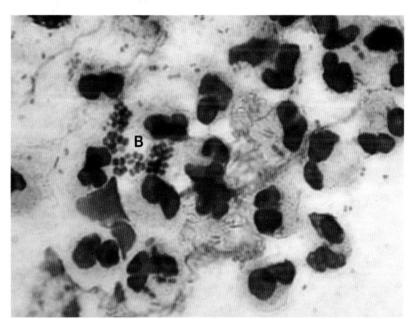

Figure 8.17 Bacterial rhinitis. Numerous neutrophils and some bacteria (B) (MGG staining; ×1000 with CMF 1.4×).

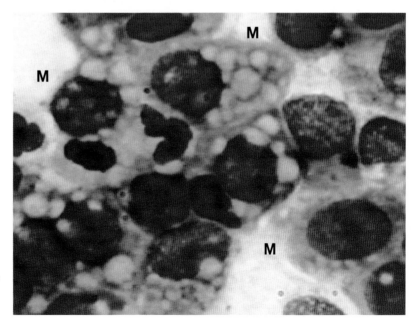

Figure 8.18 Vacuolar degeneration of metaplastic cells (M) (MGG staining; ×1000 with CMF 2.2×).

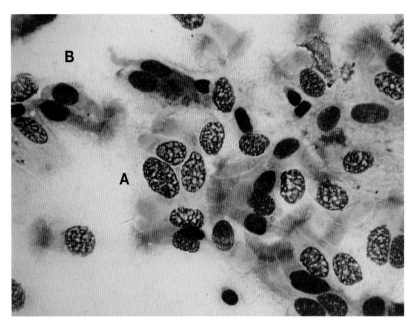

Figure 8.19 Section of nasal mucosa scraping specimen. The mature ciliated cells have a larger, less compact nucleus (A) than the new cells (B) (MGG staining; ×1000).

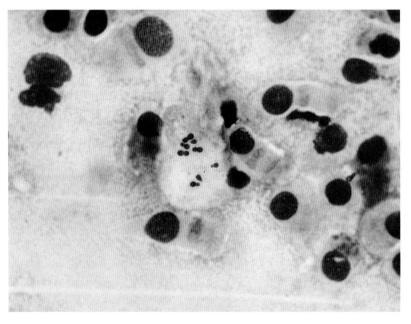

Figure 8.20 Fungal rhinitis. Spores can be seen at the center of the microscopic field (MGG staining; ×1000).

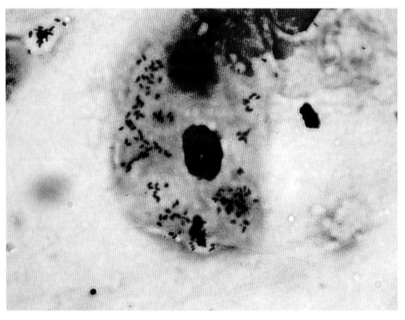

Figure 8.21 Epithelial cell of the nasal vestibule. The cell surface is covered with numerous bacteria (bacterial adhesion) (MGG staining; ×1000 with CMF 1.8×).

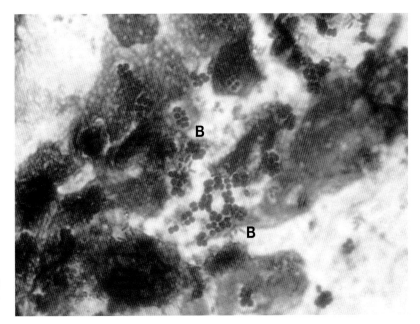

Figure 8.22 Bacterial rhinitis: numerous bacterial elements (B) appearing as "cocci" (MGG staining; ×1000 with CMF 2×).

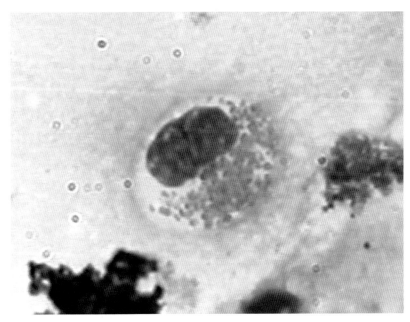

Figure 8.23 Eosinophil. Prominent acidophilic intracytoplasmic granules. The single nucleus is not bilobed as normally occurs (MGG staining; ×1000 with CMF 2×).

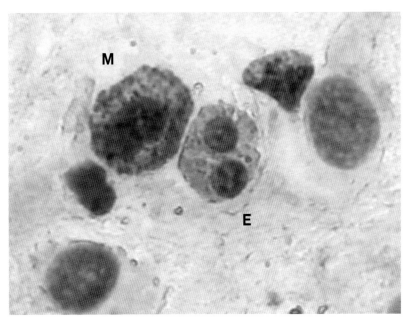

Figure 8.24 Eosinophil (E); mast cell (M) (MGG staining; ×1000 with CMF 1.4×).

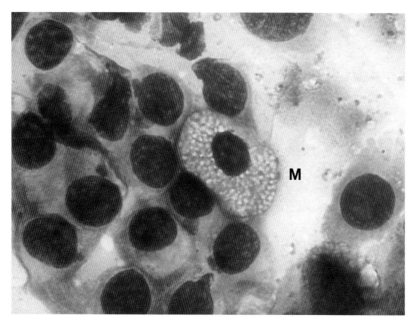

Figure 8.25 "Empty" mast cell after degranulation (M): clearly visible in the cytoplasm are numerous empty vacuoles, resulting from recent degranulation (MGG staining; ×1000 with CMF 1.2×).

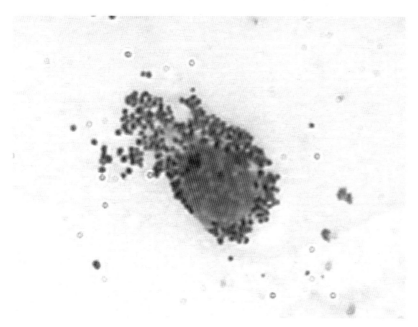

Figure 8.26 Degranulating mast cell (MGG staining; ×1000 with CMF 2×).

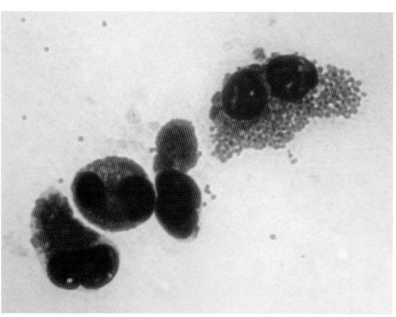

Figure 8.27 Degranulating eosinophil (MGG staining; ×1000 with CMF 2×).

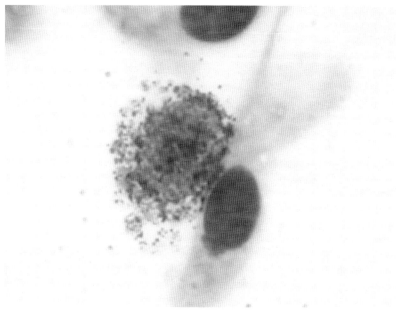

Figure 8.28 Degranulating mast cell (MGG staining; ×1000 with CMF 2×).

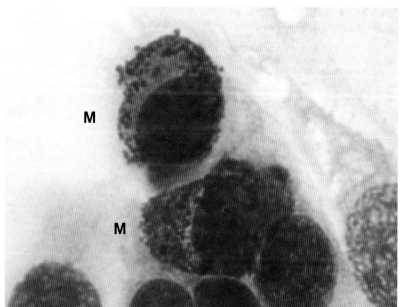

Figure 8.29 Mast cells (M) (MGG staining; ×1000 with CMF 2.2×).

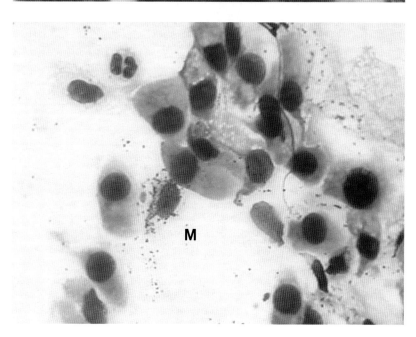

Figure 8.30 Allergic rhinitis. Degranulating mast cell (M) surrounded by metaplastic cells (MGG staining; ×1000).

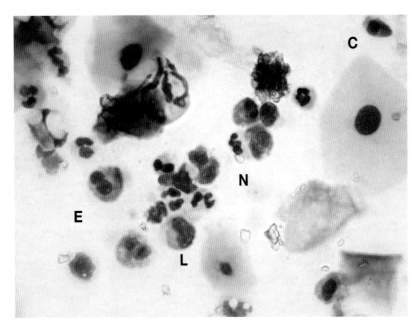

Figure 8.31 Allergic rhinitis. Eosinophils (E), neutrophil (N), lymphocyte (L), squamous cell of the nasal vestibule (nasal lavage; MGG staining; ×1000).

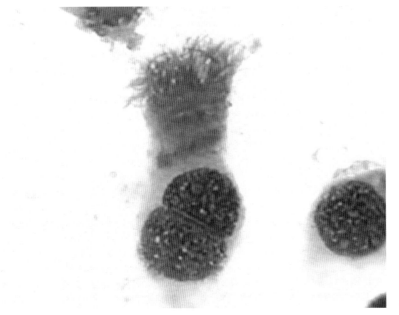

Figure 8.32 Ciliated cell with bilobed nucleus (MGG staining; ×1000 with CMF 2×).

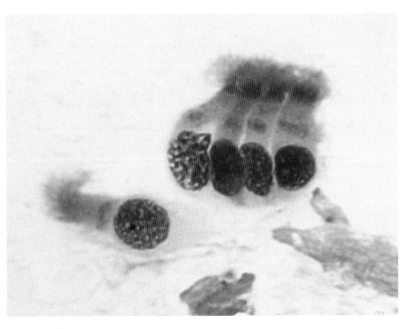

Figure 8.33 Group of ciliated cells (SHS+) (MGG staining; ×1000 with CMF 1.2×).

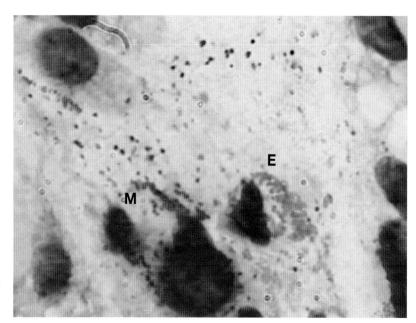

Figure 8.34 Acute phase allergic rhinitis. Massive degranulation of eosinophils and mast cells. The mast cell granules stain wine-red (M) and the eosinophils orange (E) (MGG staining; ×1000 with CMF 1.2×).

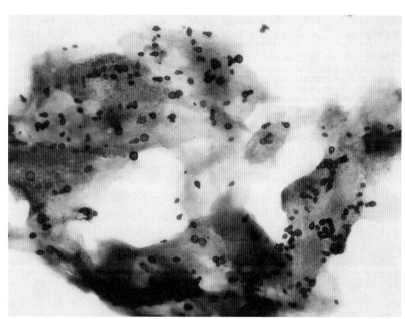

Figure 8.35 Fungal rhinitis. Colony of yeast spores, some of which are budded (MGG staining; ×1000 with CMF 1.4×).

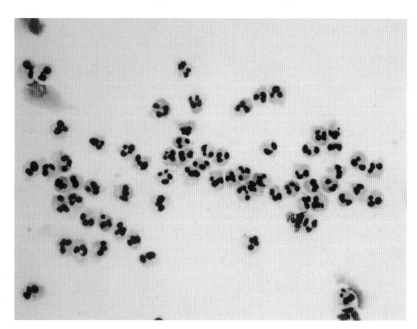

Figure 8.36 Non allergic rhinitis with neutrophils (NARNE). Group of neutrophils. Infectious agents (bacteria, fungi) are absent (MGG staining; ×1000).

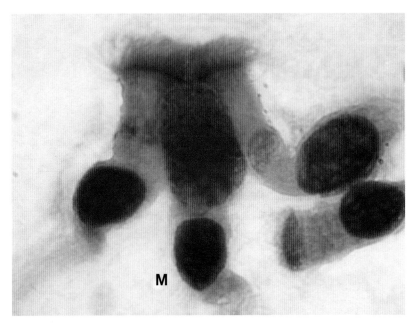

Figure 8.37 Normal cytology. Muciparous cell (M) interposed between two ciliated cells (MGG staining; ×1000 with CMF 2×).

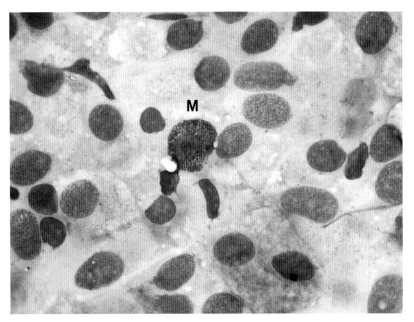

Figure 8.38 Nasal polyposis. Mast cell (M) sometimes can be mistaken for the nuclei of other cells (MGG staining; ×1000 with CMF 1.2×).

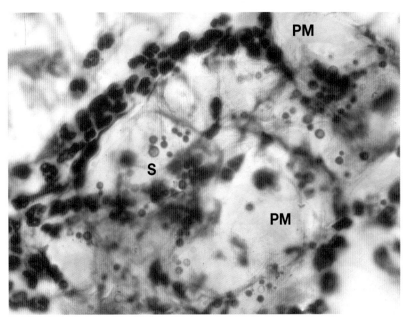

Figure 8.39 Infectious spot: numerous fungal spores (S) and rare bacteria immersed in their exopolysaccharide matrix (cyan; PM) (MGG staining; ×1000 with CMF 2.4×).

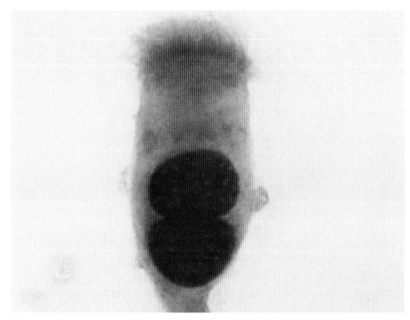

Figure 8.40 Binuclear ciliated cell (MGG staining; ×1000 with CMF 2.2×).

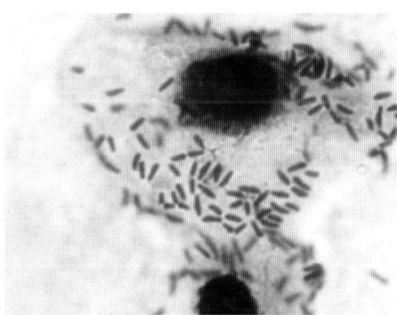

Figure 8.41 Bacterial rhinitis. Bacterial colony on epithelial cell of the nasal vestibule (MGG staining; ×1000 with CMF 4×).

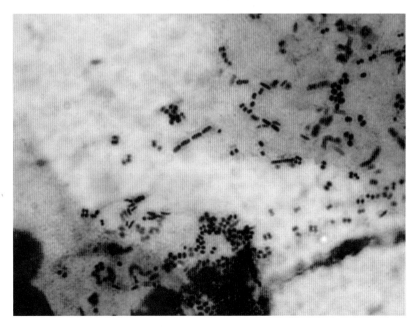

Figure 8.42 Bacterial rhinitis. Various types of bacteria (cocci, bacilli). The light "cyan" shade denotes the initial formation of biofilm (MGG staining; ×1000 with CMF 2.4×).

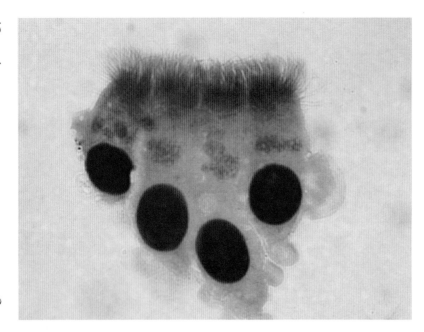

Figure 8.43 Group of ciliated cells with prominent ciliary apparatus, SHS+ (MGG staining; ×1000 with CMF 1.8×).

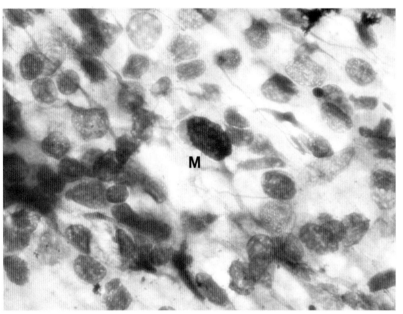

Figure 8.44 Nasal polyposis in patient with mastocytic rhinitis. Mast cell (M) at the center of an aggregate of metaplastic cells (MGG staining; ×1000).

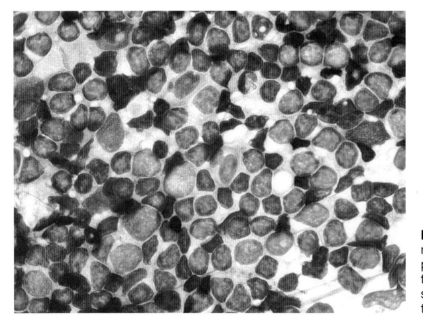

Figure 8.45 Viral infectious rhinitis: numerous lymphocytes with normal morphologic appearance of the nucleus and the cytoplasm. There are no obvious signs of cell mitosis, or discoloration of the nucleus (MGG staining; ×1000).

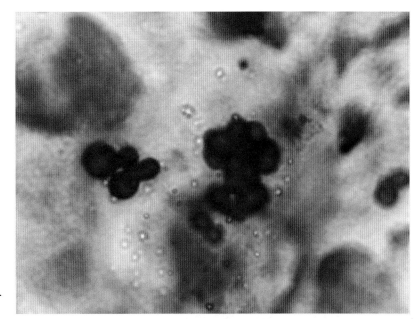

Figure 8.46 Fungal spores (MGG staining; ×1000 with CMF 4×).

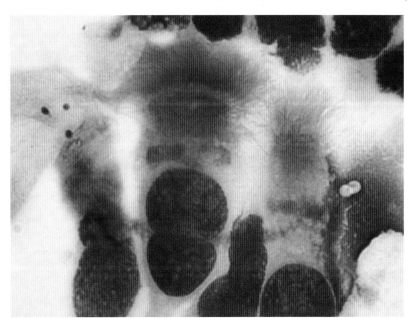

Figure 8.47 Binuclear ciliated cell. Ciliary apparatus and SHS show signs of cell regeneration (MGG staining; ×1000 with CMF 2×).

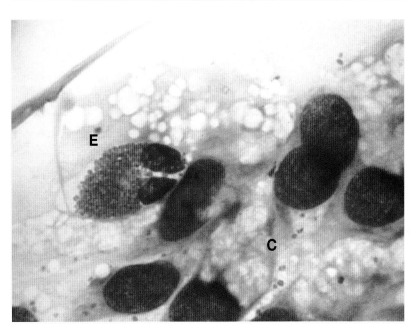

Figure 8.48 Allergic rhinitis. Eosinophil (E) with characteristic bilobed nucleus and acidophilic intracytoplasmic granules; mucous cell (C) (MGG staining; ×1000 with CMF 2.4×).

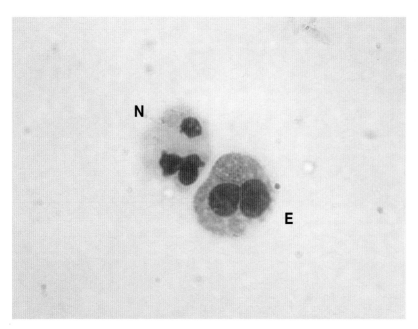

Figure 8.49 Allergic rhinitis. Differences in morphology and staining between neutrophil (N) and eosinophil (E) (MGG staining; ×1000 with CMF 2×).

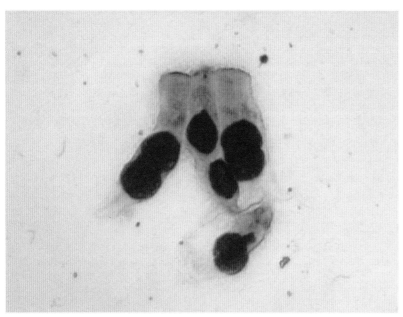

Figure 8.50 Bacterial infectious rhinitis. Binuclear ciliated cell. Dystrophic ciliary apparatus and reduction of the SHS are signs of cell damage (MGG staining; ×1000).

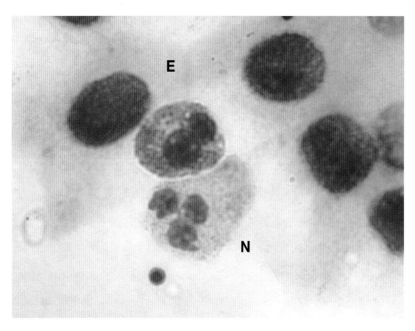

Figure 8.51 Allergic rhinitis. Differences in morphology and staining between neutrophil (N) and eosinophil (E) (MGG staining; ×1000 with CMF 2.2×).

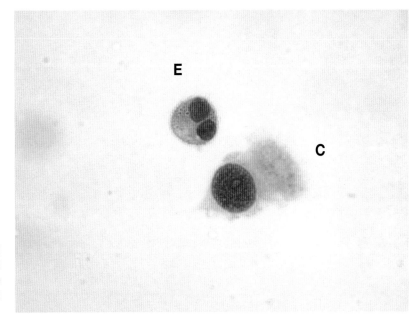

Figure 8.52 Allergic rhinitis. Eosinophil (E) with characteristic morphologic and staining features, columnar cell (C) of the nasal mucosa (MGG staining; ×1000 with CMF 1.2×).

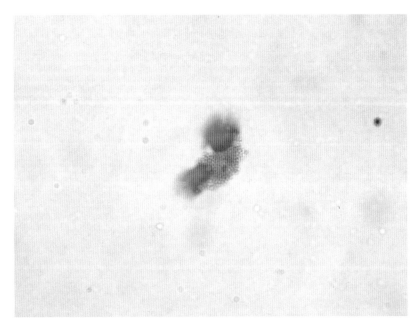

Figure 8.53 Allergic rhinitis. Disintegrated eosinophil. Staining features can sometimes help identify a cell, even when it has undergone morphologic changes during the staining process (MGG staining; ×1000 with CMF 2×).

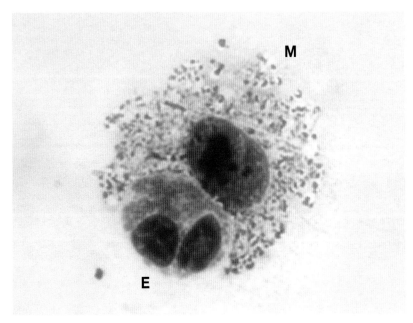

Figure 8.54 Non allergic rhinitis with eosinophils and mast cells (NARESMA): granules of a mast cell (M) encircle an eosinophil (E) (MGG staining; ×1000 with CMF 2.4×).

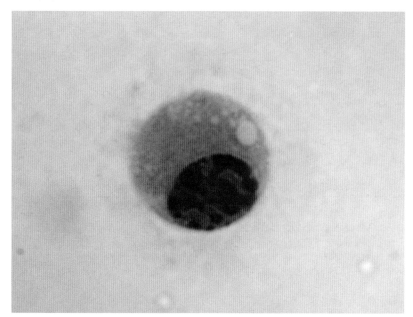

Figure 8.55 Allergic rhinitis: large lymphocyte. The increase in the cytoplasm, the appearance of intracytoplasmic vacuoles and the "tortoiseshell" nucleus indicate a process of plasma cell transformation (MGG staining; ×1000 with CMF 3.0×).

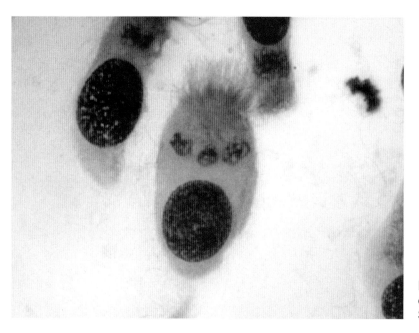

Figure 8.56 Normal cytology. Ciliated cell with prominent ciliary apparatus and SHS (MGG staining; ×1000 with CMF 2×).

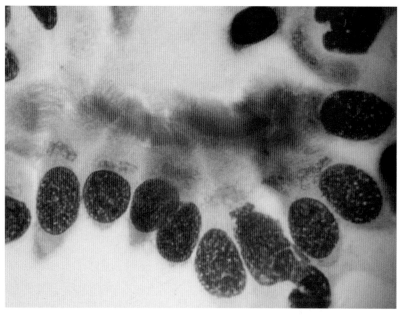

Figure 8.57 Normal cytology. Group of ciliated cells with prominent ciliary apparatus and SHS (MGG staining; ×1000 with CMF 1.4×).

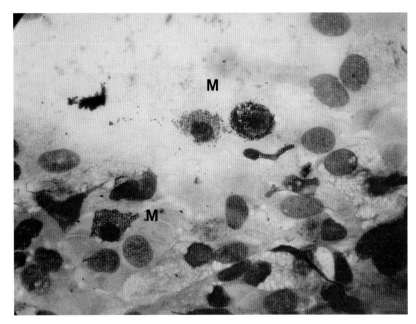

Figure 8.58 Nasal mastocytosis. Mast cells (M) (MGG staining; ×1000).

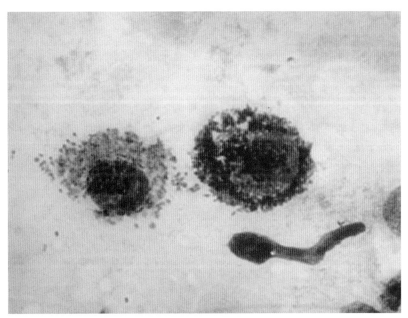

Figure 8.59 Nasal mastocytosis. Detail of Figure 8.58 at higher magnification. Mast cell granules can sometimes obscure the nucleus (MGG staining; ×1000 with CMF 2.4×).

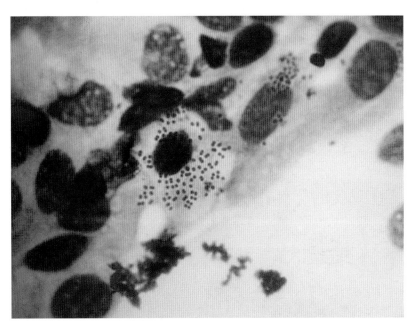

Figure 8.60 Bacterial rhinitis. Colony of coccobacilli (MGG staining; ×1000 with CMF 1.4×).

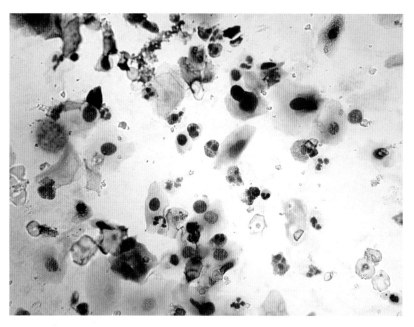

Figure 8.61 Allergic rhinitis. Numerous eosinophils and squamous cells of the nasal vestibule (nasal lavage; MGG staining; ×400).

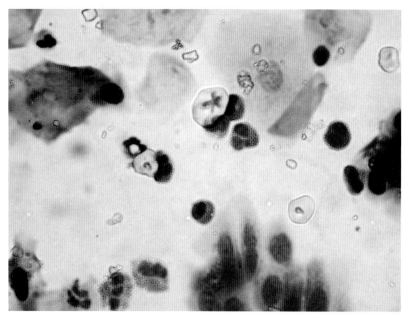

Figure 8.62 Allergic rhinitis. Same slide as in Figure 8.61 at higher magnification.

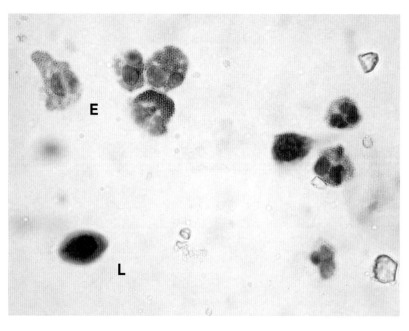

Figure 8.63 Allergic rhinitis. Eosinophils (E), activated lymphocyte (L) (nasal lavage; MGG staining; ×1000).

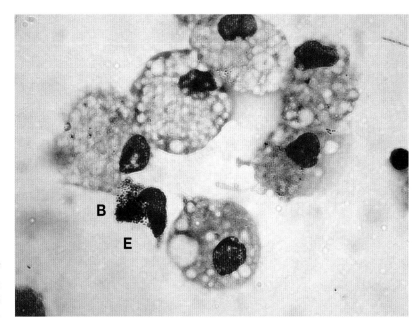

Figure 8.64 Induced sputum: a group of alveolar macrophages in a patient with bronchial asthma. Eosinophil (E); bacteria (B) (MGG staining; ×1000 with CMF 1.2×).

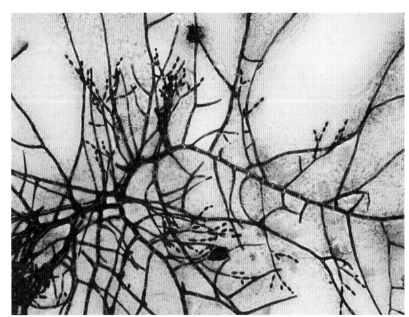

Figure 8.65 Fungal rhinitis. Candida hyphae (MGG staining; ×1000).

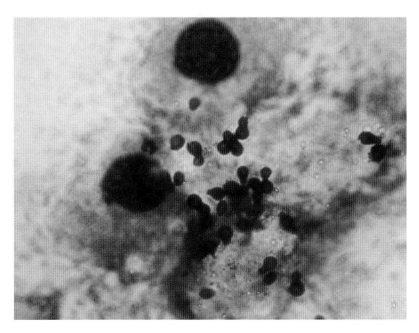

Figure 8.66 Fungal rhinitis. Yeast spores (MGG staining; ×1000 with CMF 2.4×).

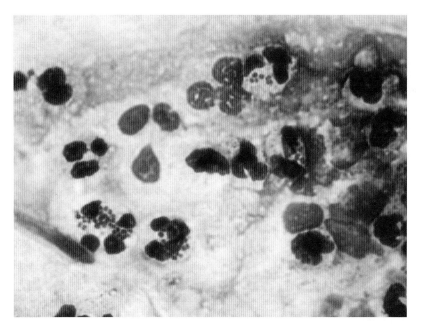

Figure 8.67 Bacterial rhinitis. Neutrophils with intracytoplasmic bacteria (MGG staining; ×1000 with CMF 1.4×).

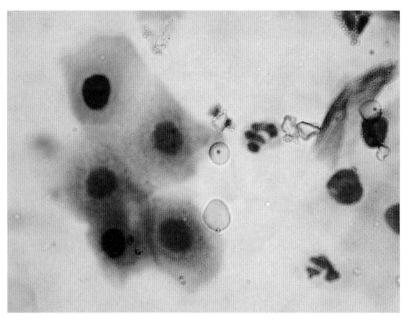

Figure 8.68 Squamous cells of the nasal vestibule (nasal lavage; MGG staining; ×1000 with CMF 1.2×).

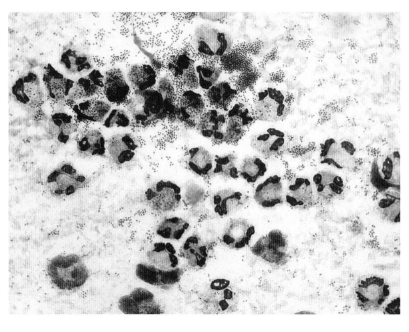

Figure 8.69 Acute rhinosinusitis: many neutrophils and bacteria, some intracellular (MGG staining; ×1000).

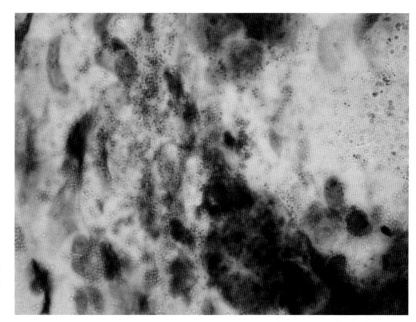

Figure 8.70 Allergic rhinitis. Massive degranulation of eosinophils. The granules stain orange with acid dyes (MGG staining; ×1000).

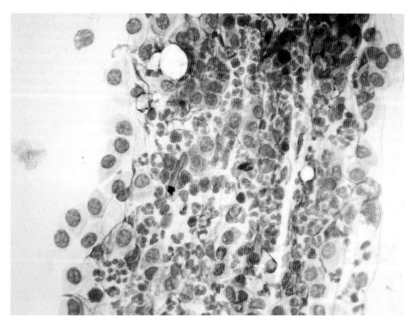

Figure 8.71 Allergic rhinitis. Numerous neutrophils and some eosinophils in nasal secretion. Eosinophils can be recognized by their reddish-orange color (MGG staining; ×400).

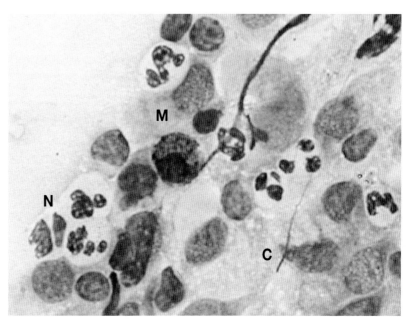

Figure 8.72 Allergic rhinitis. Mast cell (M) surrounded by neutrophils (N). Columnar cells show metaplasia (C) (MGG staining; ×1000 with CMF 1.2×).

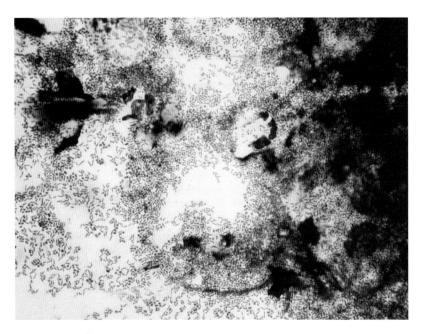

Figure 8.73 Bacterial rhinitis. Numerous bacteria and some neutrophils (MGG staining; ×1000).

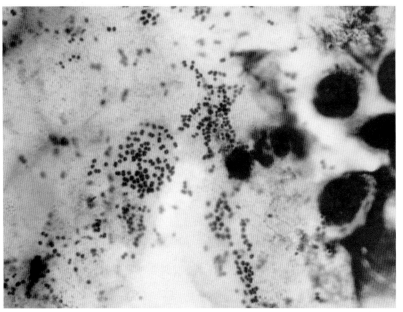

Figure 8.74 Bacterial rhinitis. Bacterial colony (MGG staining; ×1000 with CMF 1.4×).

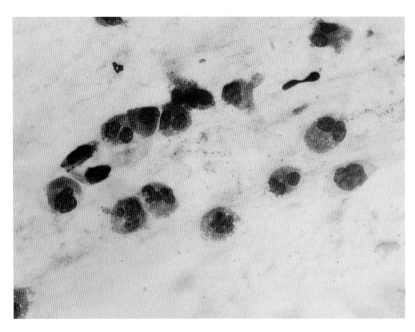

Figure 8.75 NARES. Numerous eosinophils (MGG staining; ×1000).

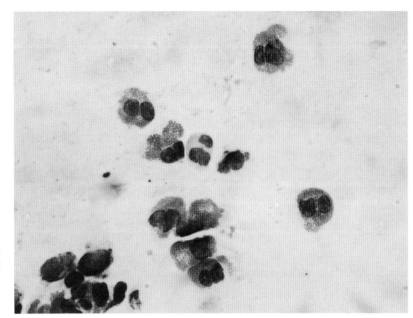

Figure 8.76 Allergic rhinitis. Eosinophils are predominant in acute phase allergic rhinitis; neutrophils are prevalent in "minimal persistent inflammation" (MGG staining; ×400).

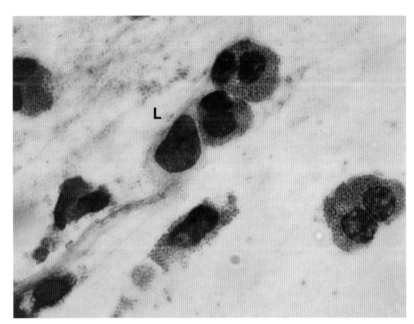

Figure 8.77 Allergic rhinitis. Eosinophils and a lymphocyte (L) at the center of the microscopic field (MGG staining; ×1000 with CMF 1.4×).

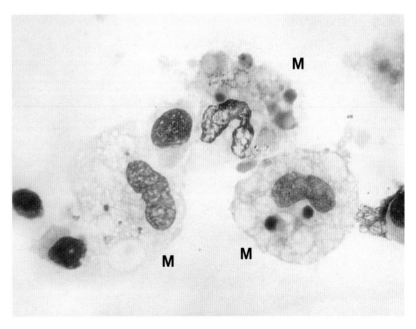

Figure 8.78 Group of macrophages (M) (MGG staining; ×1000).

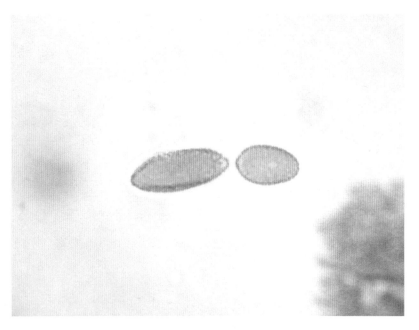

Figure 8.79 Nasal cytology: inhaled air-borne pollen (MGG staining; ×1000 with CMF 3×).

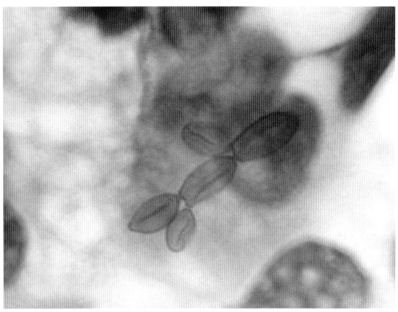

Figure 8.80 Nasal cytology: inhaled air-borne pollen (MGG staining; ×1000 with CMF 3×).

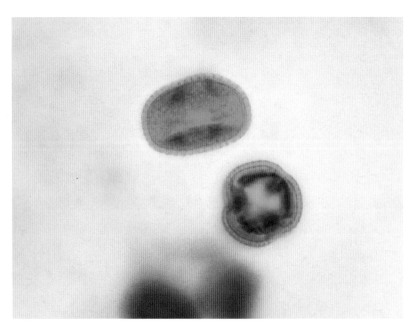

Figure 8.81 Nasal cytology: inhaled air-borne pollen (MGG staining; ×1000 with CMF 3×).

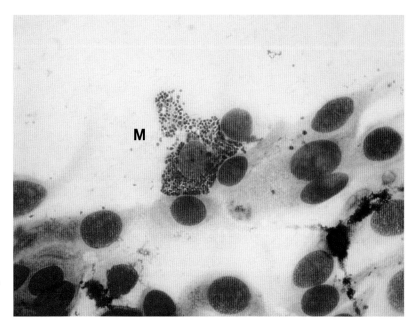

Figure 8.82 Nasal mastocytosis. Degranulated mast cell (M) (MGG staining; ×1000 with CMF 1.2×).

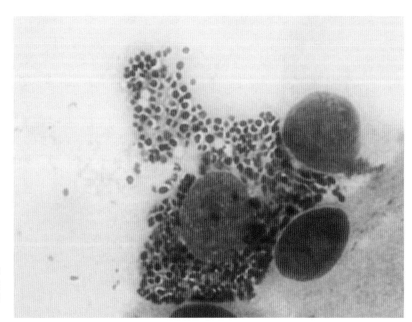

Figure 8.83 Nasal mastocytosis. Same cytological smear as in Figure 8.82 at higher magnification (MGG staining; ×1000 with CMF 4×).

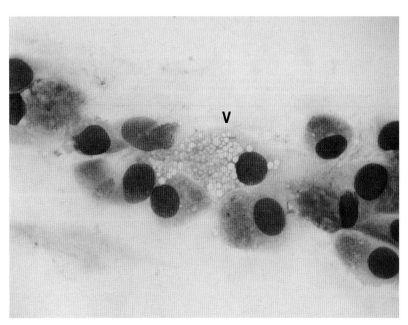

Figure 8.84 Cytoplasmic vacuoles (V) in mucous cell (MGG staining; ×1000 with CMF 1.2×).

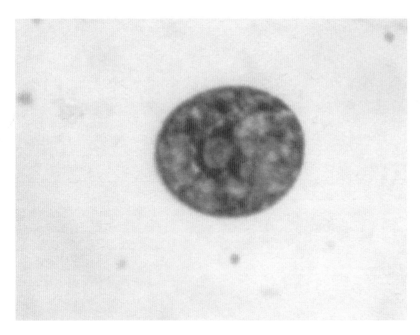

Figure 8.85 Nasal cytology: "bare" nucleus. The nucleolus (light blue) is visible inside the nucleus (MGG staining; ×1000 with CMF 3×).

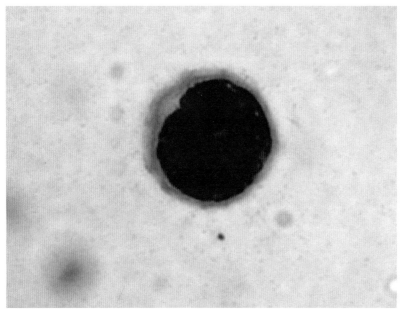

Figure 8.86 Nasal cytology: lymphocyte (MGG staining; ×1000 with CMF 4×).

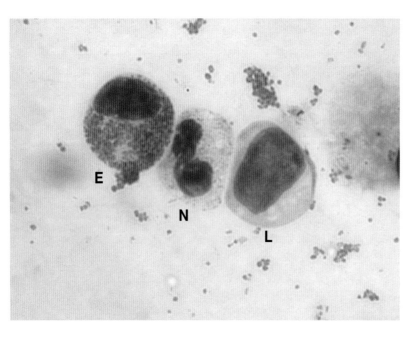

Figure 8.87 Immuno-inflammatory cells. Neutrophil (N), lymphocyte (L), eosinophil (E) (MGG staining; ×1000 with CMF 3.4×).

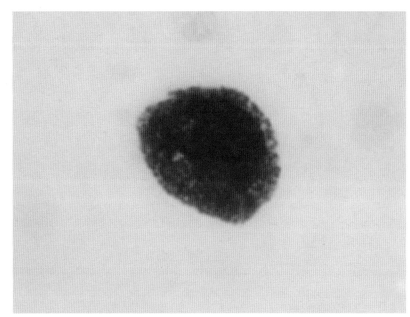

Figure 8.88 Mast cell. The compact granules obscure the cell nucleus, making it difficult to identify (MGG staining; ×1000 with CMF 3×).

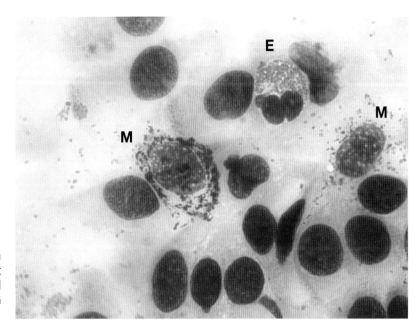

Figure 8.89 Non allergic rhinitis with eosinophil and mast cells (NARESMA). It is possible to identify eosinophils (E) and mast cells (M), partly degranulated (MGG staining; ×1000 with CMF 1.4×).

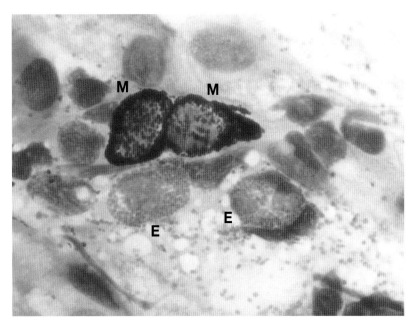

Figure 8.90 Non allergic rhinitis with eosinophils and mast cells (NARESMA). Some eosinophils (E) and mast cells (M), partly degranulated (MGG staining; ×1000 with CMF 1.8×).

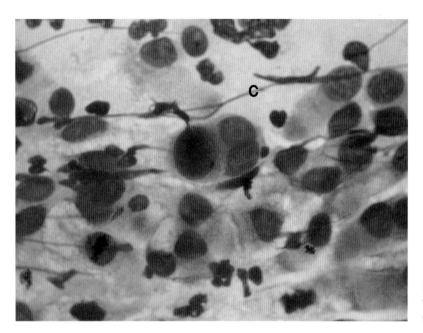

Figure 8.91 Binuclear goblet cell (C) with prominent vacuole containing mucin (MGG staining; ×1000 with CMF 1.2×).

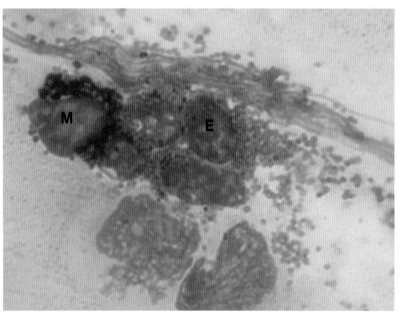

Figure 8.92 Allergic rhinitis. Degranulated eosinophil (E) and mast cell (M). Cell types can be distinguished by staining differences (MGG staining; ×1000 with CMF 3×).

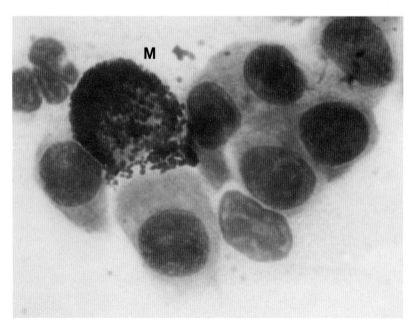

Figure 8.93 Nasal mastocytosis: mast cell (M). Basophilic granules obscure the nucleus (MGG staining; ×1000 with CMF 2.4×).

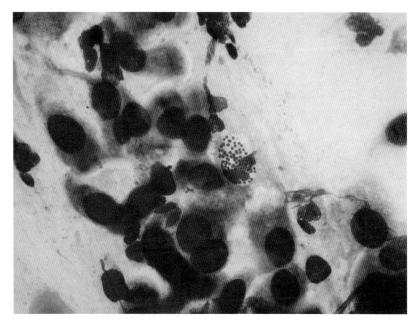

Figure 8.94 Bacterial rhinitis. Cocci bacteria phagocytized by a neutrophil (MGG staining; ×1000 with CMF 1.2×).

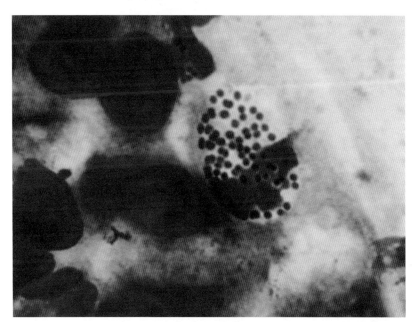

Figure 8.95 Bacterial rhinitis. Same slide as in Figure 8.94 at higher magnification (MGG staining; ×1000 with CMF 2.4×).

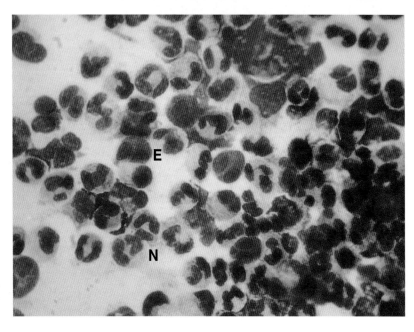

Figura 8.96 Allergic rhinitis. Numerous neutrophils (N) and scarce eosinophils (E) (MGG staining; ×1000 with CMF 1.2×).

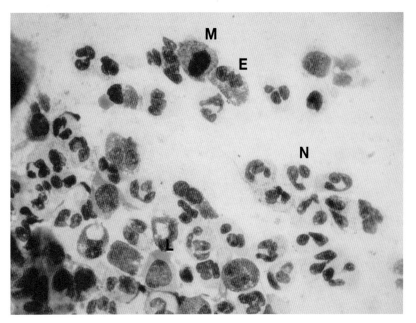

Figure 8.97 Allergic rhinitis. Numerous neutrophils (N) and scarce eosinophils (E), lymphocytes (L) and rare mast cells (M) (MGG staining; ×1000 with CMF 1.2×).

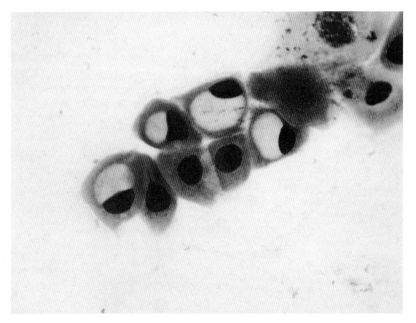

Figure 8.98 Vacuolar degeneration in a nasal mucosal cell (MGG staining; ×1000 with CMF 1.2×).

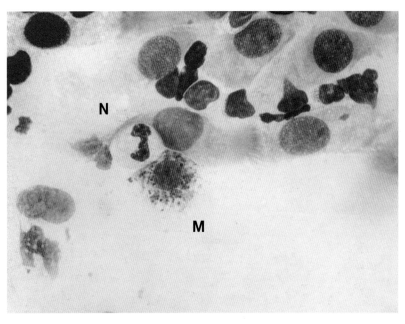

Figure 8.99 Nasal mastocytosis. Mast cell (M), neutrophil (N) (MGG staining; ×1000 with CMF 1.2×).

Figure 8.100 Fungal rhinitis. Colony of yeast spores (MGG staining; ×1000 with CMF 1.4×).

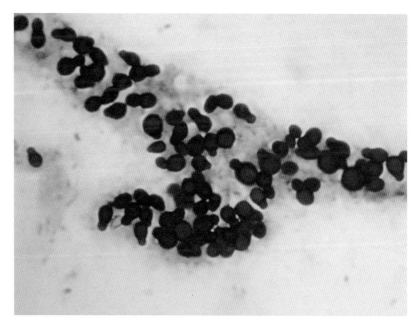

Figure 8.101 Fungal rhinitis. Colony of yeast spores (MGG staining; ×1000 with CMF 3×).

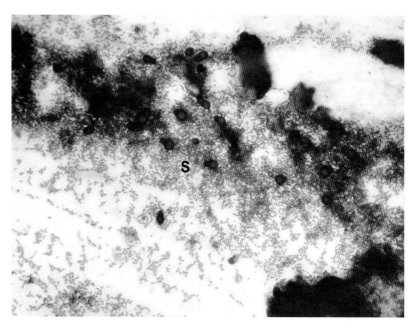

Figure 8.102 Bacterial rhinitis with fungal superinfection. Fungal spores (S) (MGG staining; ×1000 with CMF 1.4×).

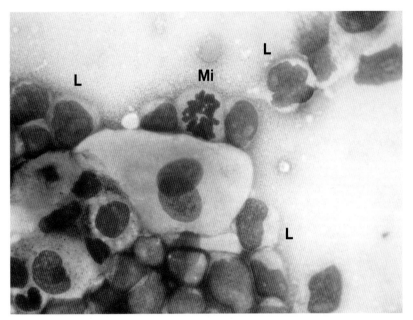

Figure 8.103 Nasal lymphoma: numerous lymphocytes (L) with alterations of the nucleus (discoloration, signs of mitosis [Mi], etc.) and of the cytoplasm (MGG staining; ×1000 with CMF 1.8×).

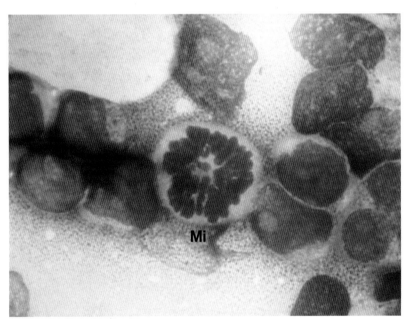

Figure 8.104 Nasal lymphoma: a lymphocyte undergoing mitosis (Mi) (MGG staining; ×1000 with CMF 2.2×).

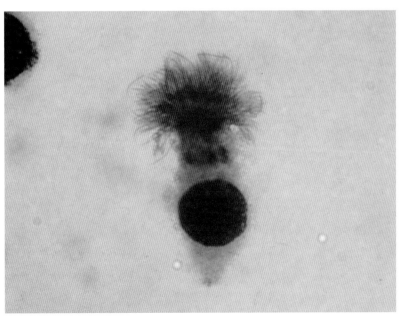

Figure 8.105 Ciliated cell. Prominent ciliary apparatus and SHS (MGG staining; ×1000 with CMF 1.8×).

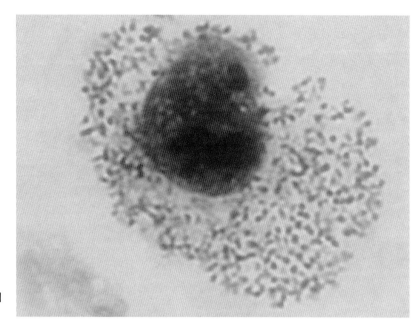

Figure 8.106 Degranulating mast cell (MGG staining; ×1000 with CMF 4×).

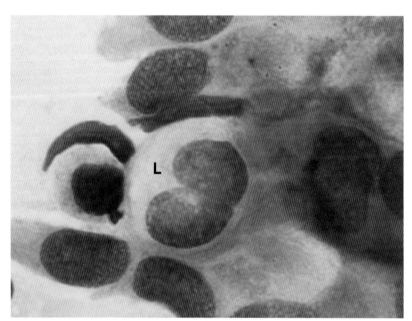

Figure 8.107 Large lymphocyte (L) (MGG staining; ×1000 with CMF 2.8×).

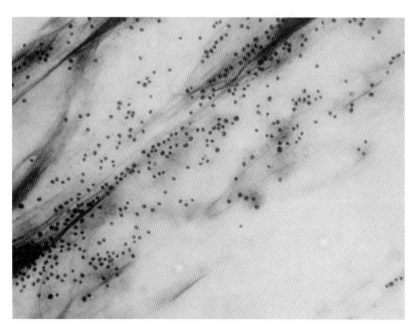

Figure 8.108 Bacterial rhinitis (MGG staining; ×1000 with CMF 1.2×).

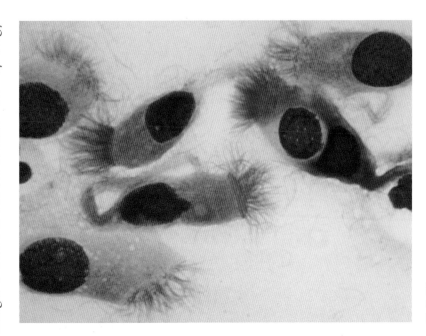

Figure 8.109 Cell with well-defined ciliary apparatus (MGG staining; ×1000 with CMF 1.4×).

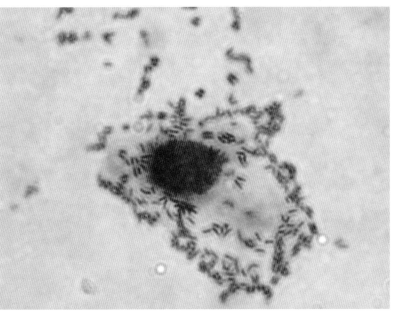

Figure 8.110 Bacteria adhering to a squamous cell of the nasal vestibule (MGG staining; ×1000 with CMF 2.2×).

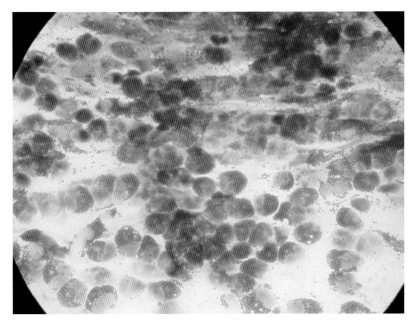

Figure 8.111 Nasal polyposis: numerous eosinophils, mainly degranulated (MGG staining; ×1000).

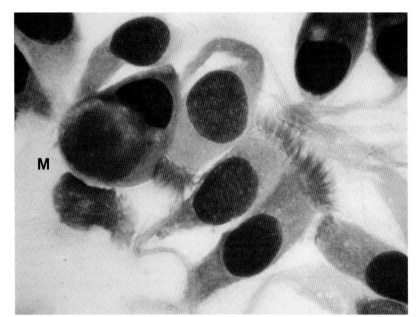

Figure 8.112 Caliciform mucous (goblet) cell (M), ciliated cells. SHS– (MGG staining; ×1000 with CMF 1.4×).

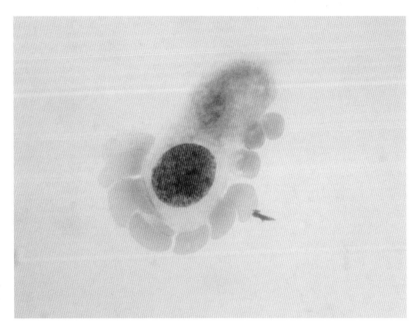

Figure 8.113 Nasal scraping specimen. Columnar cell of the nasal mucosa surrounded by erythrocytes (MGG staining; ×1000 with CMF 1.4×).

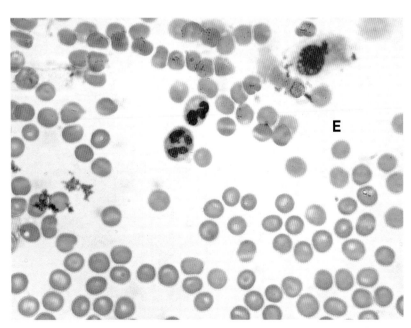

Figure 8.114 Nasal scraping specimen. Numerous erythrocytes (E) on the nasal cytogram is often a sign of incorrect sampling (MGG staining; ×400).

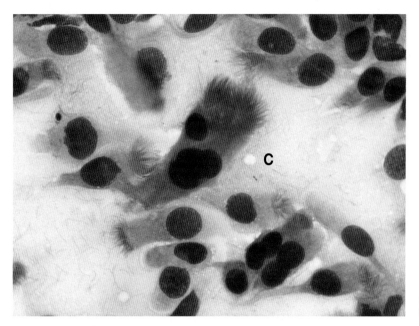

Figure 8.115 Polynuclear cell (C) (MGG staining; ×1000).

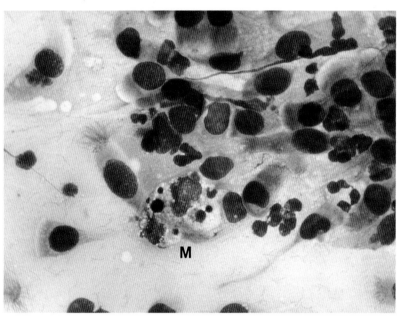

Figure 8.116 Macrophage (M) with cytoplasm filled with phagocytotic products (MGG staining; ×1000).

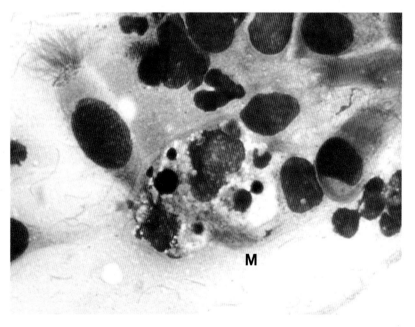

Figure 8.117 Same slide as in Figure 8.116 at higher magnification (MGG staining; ×1000 with CMF 1.2×).

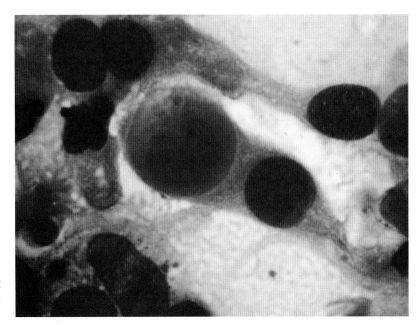

Figure 8.118 Goblet cell. Prominent vacuole containing intracytoplasmic mucin (MGG staining; ×1000 with CMF 2×).

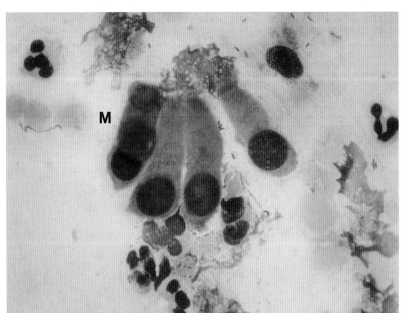

Figure 8.119 Ciliated columnar cells, mucous cells (M) and some neutrophils (MGG staining; ×1000).

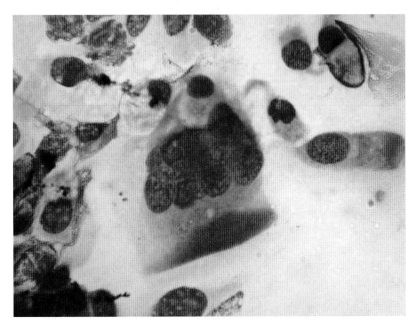

Figure 8.120 Viral rhinitis. Large columnar cell of the nasal epithelium showing polynucleation. Prominent nucleoli inside the nuclei (MGG staining; ×1000).

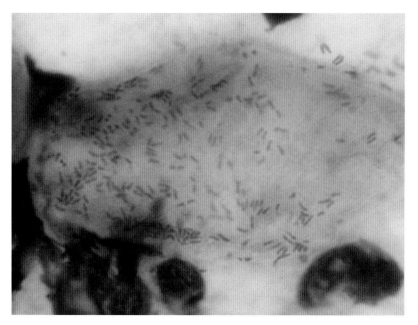

Figure 8.121 Infectious spot. Numerous bacteria embedded in a exopolysaccharide matrix (morphologic-chromatic expression of biofilm) (MGG staining; ×1000 with CMF 1.2×).

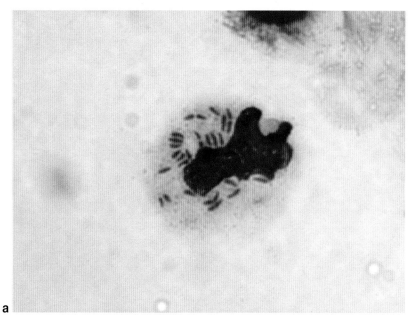

a

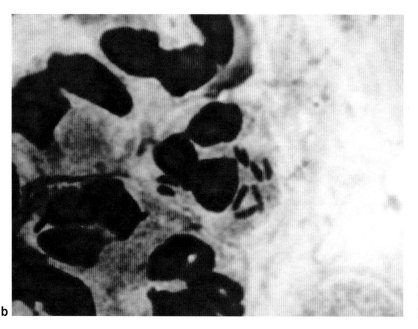

b

Figure 8.122 a-b Neutrophil with numerous phagocytized intracellular bacteria (MGG staining; ×1000 with CMF 4×).

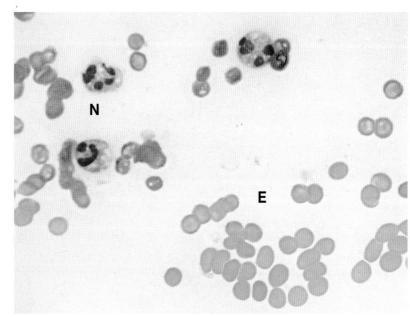

Figure 8.123 Numerous erythrocytes (E) and some neutrophils (N) (MGG staining; ×1000).

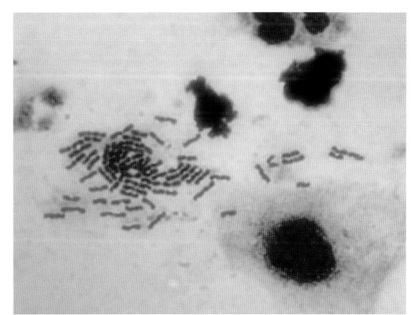

Figure 8.124 Bacterial rhinitis. Colony of bacteria (MGG staining; ×1000 with CMF 2.8×).

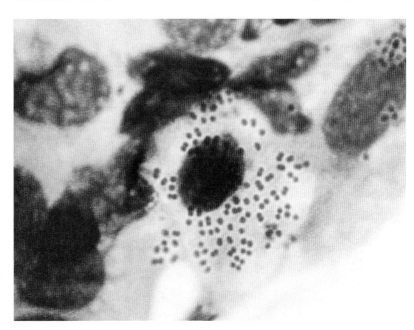

Figure 8.125 Bacterial rhinitis. Numerous bacteria are localized at epithelial cell surface of nasal vestibule (MGG staining; ×1000 with CMF 2.8×).

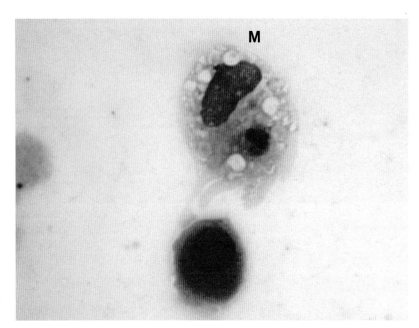

Figure 8.126 Macrophage (M). Kidney-shaped nucleus and cytoplasm containing numerous vacuoles and phagosomes (MGG staining; ×1000 with CMF 1.2×).

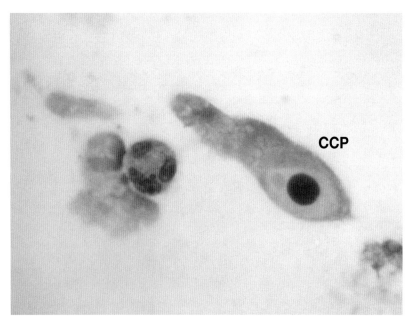

Figure 8.127 Viral rhinitis: cell with clear signs of ciliocytophthoria (MGG staining; ×1000 with CMF 1.4×).

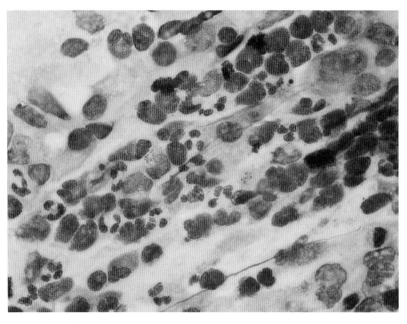

Figure 8.128 Acute phase allergic rhinitis. Eosinophils, neutrophils, lymphocytes (MGG staining; ×1000).

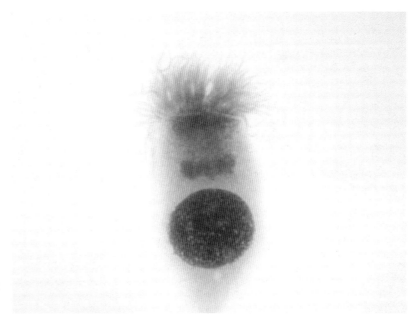

Figure 8.129 Ciliated cell with prominent supranuclear hyperchromatic stria (SHS+) (MGG staining; ×1000 with CMF 2×).

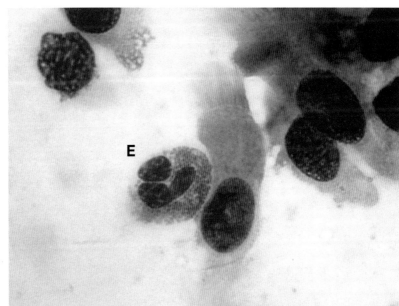

Figure 8.130 Eosinophil with trilobed nucleus (E) next to a SHS– ciliated cell (MGG staining; ×1000 with CMF 1.4×).

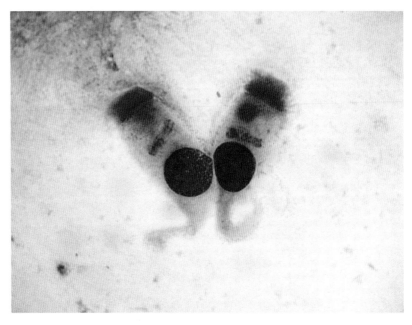

Figure 8.131 Prominent SHS+ ciliated cell (MGG staining; ×1000 with CMF 1.2×).

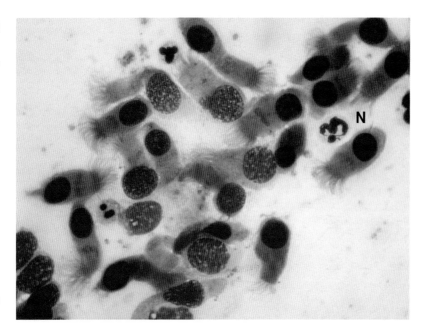

Figure 8.132 Normal nasal cytogram with SHS+ ciliated cells and sporadic neutrophils (N) (MGG staining; ×1000).

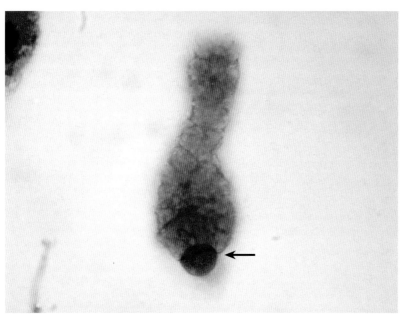

Figure 8.133 Goblet cell with condensed nuclear chromatin (arrow) (MGG staining; ×1000 with CMF 1.8×).

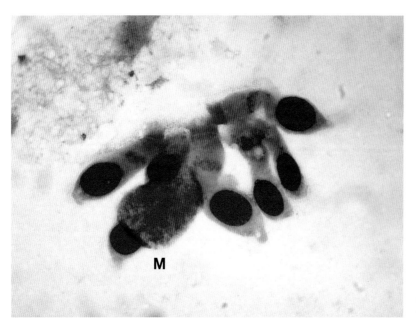

Figure 8.134 Ciliated cells and mucous cell (M) in characteristic ratio of 4 ciliated to 1 goblet cell (MGG staining; ×1000).

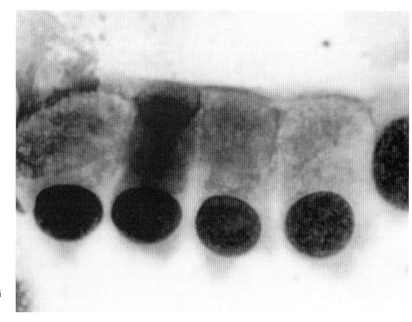

Figure 8.135 Group of striate cells (MGG staining; ×1000 with CMF 2×).

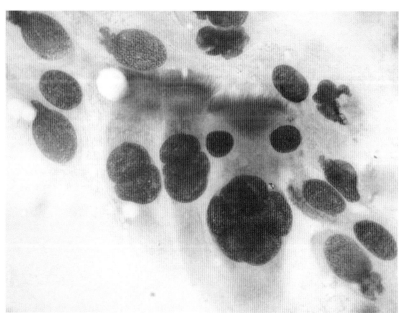

Figure 8.136 Multinuclear ciliated cells (MGG staining; ×1000 with CMF 1.2×).

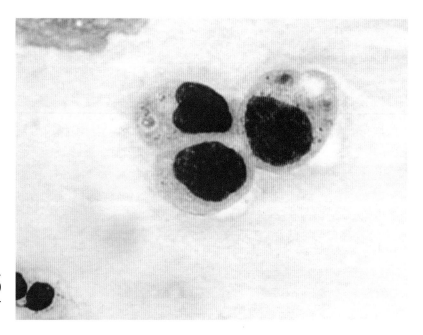

Figure 8.137 Group of lymphocytes. Small granulations stained red (lysosomes) are evident in the cytoplasm (MGG staining; ×1000 with CMF 2×).

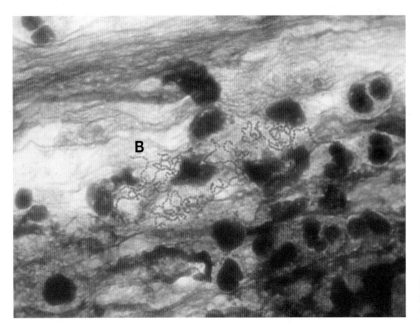

Figure 8.138 Bacterial rhinitis: streptococcus bacteria (B) (MGG staining; ×1000 with CMF 1.2×).

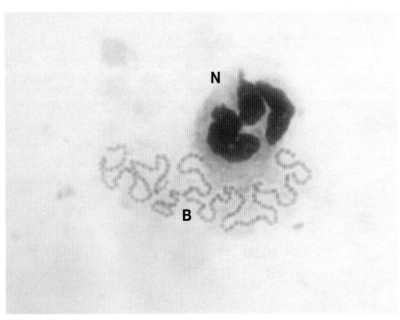

Figure 8.139 Bacterial rhinitis: streptococcus bacteria (B) at higher magnification and neutrophil (N) (MGG staining; ×1000 with CMF 1.8×).

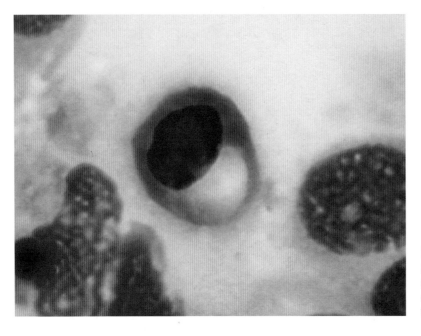

Figure 8.140 Plasma cell. Immunoglobulins are produced in the sarcoplasm, a slightly pale area of the cytoplasm adjacent to the nucleus (MGG staining; ×1000 with CMF 2.2×).

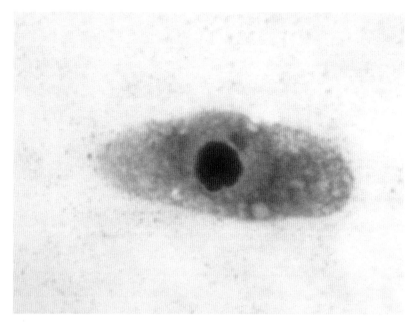

Figure 8.141 Viral rhinitis: cell with signs of ciliocytophthoria (MGG staining; ×1000 with CMF 2×).

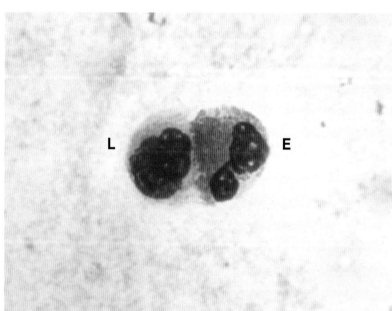

Figure 8.142 Lymphocyte (L) adhering to an eosinophil (E) (MGG staining; ×1000 with CMF 1.4×).

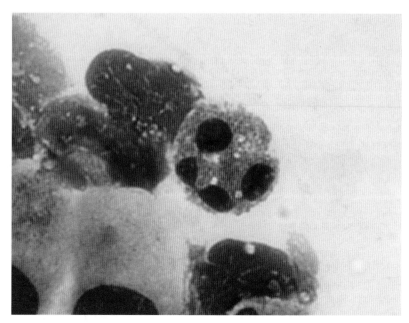

Figure 8.143 Eosinophil with quadrilobated nucleus (MGG staining; ×1000 with CMF 1.8×).

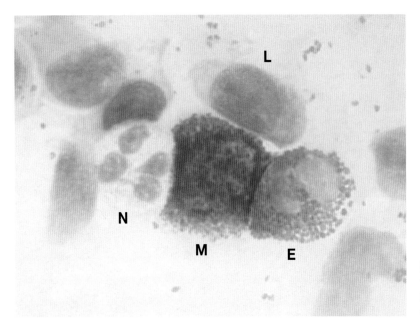

Figure 8.144 Inflammatory cells: neutrophil (N), mast cell (M), eosinophil (E), lymphocyte (L) (MGG staining; ×1000 with CMF 1.8×).

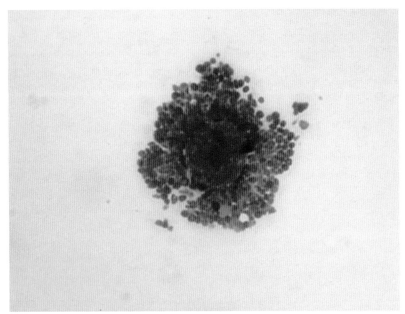

Figure 8.145 Degranulating mast cell (MGG staining; ×1000 with CMF 1.8×).

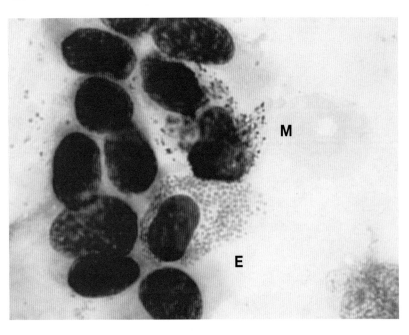

Figure 8.146 Degranulating eosinophil (E) and mast cell (M) in a patient affected by NARESMA (MGG staining; ×1000 with CMF 1.4×).

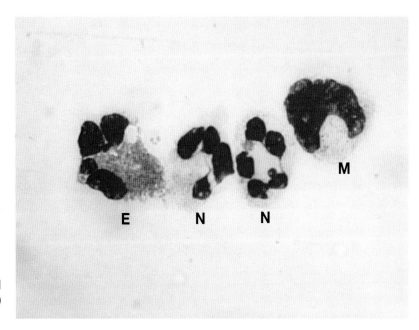

Figure 8.147 Group of cells: eosinophil (E), neutrophils (N) and monocyte (M) (MGG staining; ×1000 with CMF 1.4×).

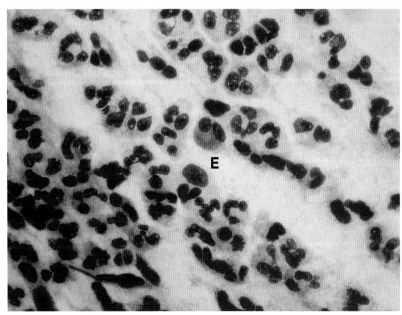

Figure 8.148 Dust mite-sensitive allergic rhinitis. Numerous neutrophils surrounding an eosinophil (E) (minimal persistent inflammation) (MGG staining; ×1000).

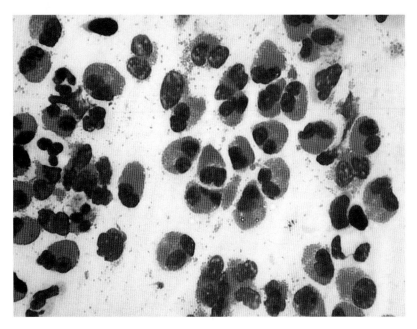

Figure 8.149 Non allergic rhinitis with eosinophilia syndrome (NARES). Prevalence of eosinophils (MGG staining; ×1000 with CMF 1.2×).

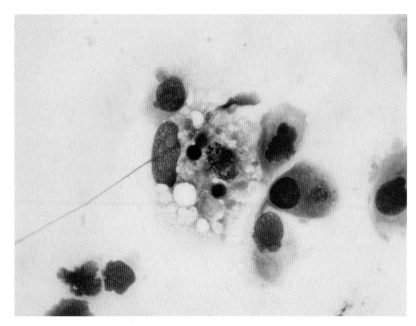

Figure 8.150 Macrophage. Oval nucleus with prominent nucleolus and cytoplasm with numerous vacuoles and inclusions (MGG staining; ×1000).

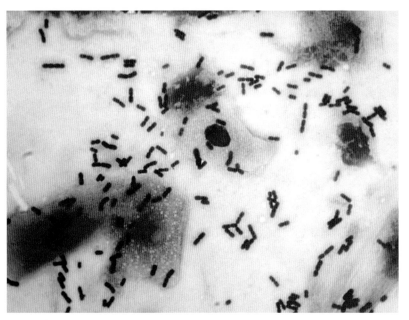

Figure 8.151 Bacterial infectious rhinitis. Pneumococcal bacteria (MGG staining; ×1000 with CMF 2.8×).

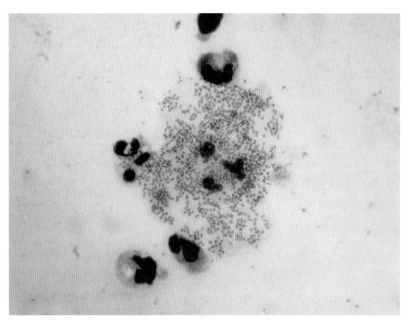

Figure 8.152 Bacterial infectious rhinitis. Bacterial colony and neutrophil chemotaxis (MGG staining; ×1000).

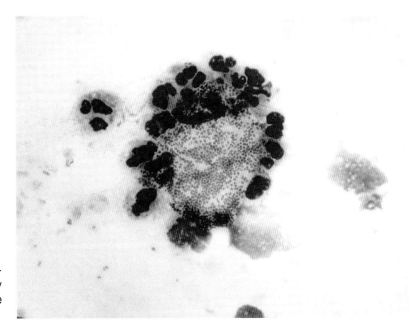

Figure 8.153 Bacterial infectious rhinitis. Numerous neutrophils, attracted by chemotactic factors, have encircled the bacterial colony (MGG staining; ×1000).

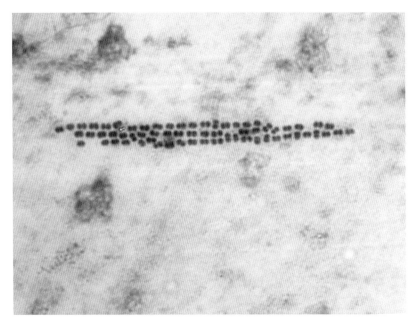

Figure 8.154 Streptococcal bacteria (MGG staining; ×1000 with CMF 2.8×).

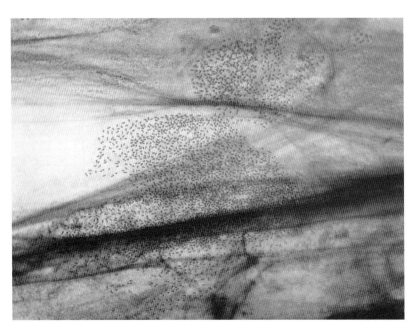

Figure 8.155 Pneumococcal colony. The halo around the bacterium is the bacterial capsule (MGG staining; ×1000).

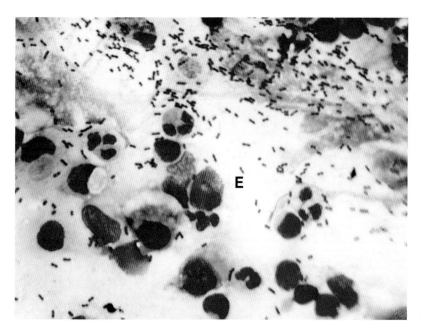

Figure 8.156 Allergic rhinitis with bacterial superinfection. Eosinophil (E) (MGG staining; ×1000 with CMF 1.2×).

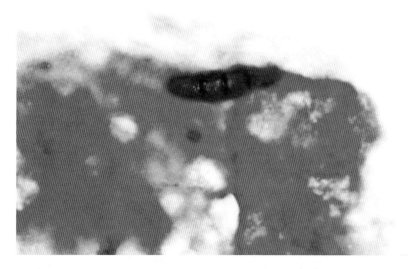

Figure 8.157 Fungal rhinitis. *Alternaria* spores (MGG staining; ×1000 with CMF 3×).

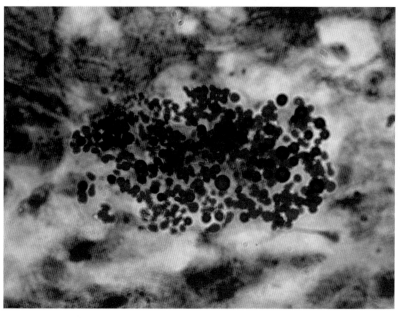

Figure 8.158 Fungal rhinitis. Spore colony (MGG staining; ×1000 with CMF 3×).

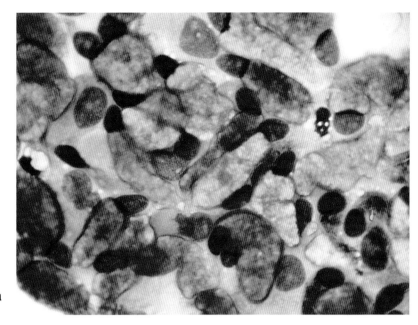

Figure 8.159 Muciparous metaplasia (MGG staining; ×1000 with CMF 1.2×).

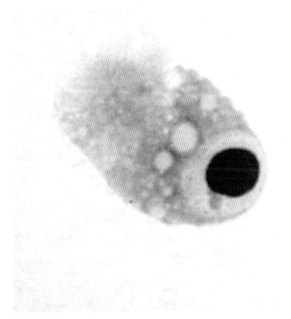

Figure 8.160 Viral rhinitis. Ciliated cell showing evidence of ciliocytophthoria (MGG staining; ×1000 with CMF 2×).

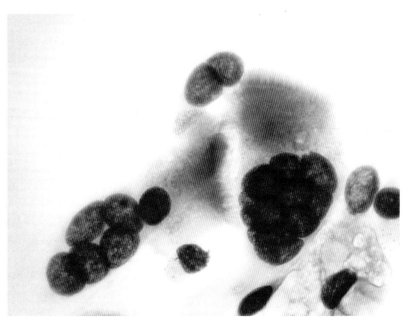

Figure 8.161 Viral rhinitis. Cells showing evidence of multinucleation (MGG staining; ×1000 with CMF 1.8×).

References

Advanced Laboratory Methods in Histology and Pathology. Washington, DC: Armed Forces Institute of Pathology American Registry of Pathology, 1994.

ANGEL-SOLANO G, SHTURMAN R. Comparative cytology of nasal secretions and nasal mucosa in allergic rhinitis. Ann Allergy 1986, 56-521.

ANDERSON HA. Practical nasal cytology: key to the problem nose. J.C.E.O.R.L. and Allergy 1979; January.

ANTONELLI A, BISETTI A, FERRARA A et al. Fisiologia e fisiopatologia del tratto respiratorio integrato. Milano: Edizioni Scientifiche Valeas, 1995.

BAIARDINI I, BRAIDO F, BRANDI S, CANONICA GW. Allergic diseases and their impact on quality of life. Ann Allergy Asthma Immunol. 2006; 97: 419-28.

BESIS M. Reinterpretation des frottis sanguins. Berlin Heidelberg: Springer-Verlag, 1980.

BICKMORE JT. Nasal cytology in allergy and infection. Otorhinolaryngology Allergy 1978; 40: 39-46.

BOGAERTS P, CLEMENT P. The diagnostic value of a cytogram in rhinopathology. Rhinology 1981; 19: 203-8.

BONIFAZI F. La diagnosi di allergia e la diagnosi di malattia. In Trattato Italiano di Allergologia, Cap. 21. Pavia: Selecta Medica, 389-437, 2002.

BOUSQUET J, KALTHAEV N, DENBURG J et al. Allergic Rhinitis and its Impact on Asthma (ARIA) 2008 update (in collaboration with the World Health Organization, GA(2) LEN and AllerGen). Allergy 2008; 63(Suppl 86): 8-160.

BOYSEN M, ZADIG E, DIGERNE V et al. Nasal mucosa in workers exposed to formaldehyde: a pilot study. Br J Indust Med 1990; 47: 116-21.

BREUER R, ZAIJCEK G, CHRISTENSEN TG, LUCEY EC, SNIDER GL. Cell kinetics of normal adult hamster bronchial epithelium in the steady state. Am J Respir Cell Mol Biol 1990; 2: 51-8.

BROWDEN DH. Cell turnover in the lung. Am Rev Respir Dis 1983; 128: S46-S48.

BRYAN MP, BRYAN WTK. Cytologic diagnosis in allergic disorders. Otolaryngol Clin North Am 1974; 7: 637-66.

BRYAN MP. BRYAN WTK, SMITH CA. Human ciliated epithelial cells in nasal secretion. Morphologic and histochemical aspect. Ann Otol Rhinol Laryngol 1964; 73: 474.

BRYAN WTK, BRYAN MT. Cytologic diagnosis in otolaryngology. Trans Am Acad Ophthalmol Otolaryngol 1959; 63: 597-611.

CARPAGNANO GE, CARRATÚ P, GELARDI M et al. Increased IL-6 and IL-4 in exhaled breath condensate of patients with nasal polyposis. MP. Monaldi Arch Chest Dis. 2009 Mar; 71(1): 3-7.

CARPAGNANO GE, RESTA O, GELARDI M et al. Exhaled inflammatory markers in aspirin-induced asthma syndrome. Am J Rhinol 2007 Sep-Oct; 21: 542-7.

CARUSO G, GELARDI M, PASSALI GC, DE SANTI MM. Nasal scraping in diagnosing ciliary dyskinesia. Am J Rhinol. 2007 Nov-Dec; 21(6): 702-5.

CASSANO M, CASSANO P, LUIGI M, GELARDI M, FARRÀS AC, FIORELLA ML. Rhino-bronchial syndrome in children: pathogenic correlations and clinical-experimental aspects. Int J Pediatr Otorhinolaryngol. 2006 Mar; 70(3): 507-13.

CASTANO P. Digital photography through the light microscope. Milano: Nikon Editor, 2000.

CHAPELIN C, COSTE A, GILAIN L, PORON F, VERRA F, ESCUDIER E. Modified epithelial cell distribution in chronic airways inflammation. Eur Respir J 1996; 9: 2474-8.

CIPRANDI G, BUSCAGLIA S, PESCE G et al. Minimal persistent inflammation is present at mucosal level in patients with asymptomatic rhinitis and mite allergy. J Allergy Clin Immunol 1995; 96: 971-9.

COHEN GA, MACPHERSON GA, GOLEMBESKY HE et al. Normal nasal cytology in infancy. Ann Allergy 1985; 54: 112-24.

CONNELL JT. Nasal Mastocytosis. J Allergy 1969; 43: 182.

COSTE A, RATEAU JG, CHAPELIN C et al. Epithelial cell proliferation in inflammatory respiratory mucosa. Am J Respir Crit Care Med 1994; 149: 992.

DALLEGRI F, OTTONELLO L. L'infiammazione delle vie aeree. Milano: EUCOS Editore, 1992.

DAVIES DG. Understanding biofilm resistance to antibacterial agents. Nature 2003; 2: 114-22.

DE PHILLIPS F. Tinuing Medical Education Series Hospital Infections. London: IPC - Science e Medicine, 1999.

ELLIS AK, KEITH PK. Nonallergic rhinitis with eosinophilia syndrome and related disorders. Clin Allergy Immunol. 2007; 19: 87-100.

EVANS MJ, PLOPPER GG. The role of basal cells in adhesion of columnar epithelium to airway basement membrane. Am Rev Respir Dis 1988; 138: 481.

EYERMANN CH. Nasal manifestations of allergy. Ann Otol; 1927; 36: 808-15.

FERGUSON BJ, STOLZ DB. Demonstration of biofilm in human bacterial chronic rhinosinusitis. Am J Rhinol. 2005; 19(5): 452-7.

FOKKENS W, LUND V, BACHERT C et al. EAACI position paper on rhinosinusitis and nasal polyps executive summary. Allergy 2005; 60: 583-601.

FRATI L. Biologia cellulare. Lederl Ocology Training Programma 1987; Volume 14, Supplemento 3.

GALINDO C, JALOWAYSKI A, MELTZER E. Correlation between nasal cytogram and blown technique for the diagnosis of allergic rhinitis. Ann Allergy 1991; 66: 86.

GANDERTON L, CHAWLA J, WINTERS C, WIMPENNY J, STICKLER D. Scanning electron microscopy of bacterial biofilms on indwelling bladder catheters. Eur J Clin Microbiol Infect Dis. 1992; 11(9): 789-96.

GARAY R. Mechanisms of vasomotor rhinitis. Allergy 2004; 59(Suppl 76): 4-9.

GELARDI M, CASSANO P, CASSANO M, FIORELLA ML. Nasal cytology: description of a hyperchromatic supranuclear stria as a possible marker for the anatomical and functional integrity of the ciliated cell. American Journal of Rhinology 2003; 17(5): 263-8.

GELARDI M, TOMAIUOLO M, CASSANO M, BESOZZI G, FIORELLA ML, CALVARIO A, CASTELLANO MA, CASSANO P. Epstein-Barr virus induced cellular changes in nasal mucosa. Virol J 2006 Feb 1; 3: 6.

GELARDI M, MASELLI DEL GIUDICE A, CANDREVA T, FIORELLA ML, ALLEN M, KLERSY C, MARSEGLIA GL, CIPRANDI G. Nasal resistance and allergic inflammation depend on allergen type. Int Arch Allergy Immunol 2006; 141(4): 384-9.

GELARDI M, FIORELLA ML, LEO G, INCORVAIA C. Cytology in the diagnosis of rhinosinusitis. Pediatr Allergy Immunol. 2007; 18 (Suppl.18): 50-2.

GELARDI M, MASELLI DEL GIUDICE A et al. Quality of life in non-allergic rhinitis depends on the predominant inflammatory cell type. J Biol Regul Homeost Agents 2008; 22: 73-81.

GELARDI M, MASELLI DEL GIUDICE A et al. Non-allergic rhinitis with eosinophils and mast cells (NARESMA) constitutes a new severe nasal disorder. Int Journal Immunopathol Pharmacolol. 2008; 23: 325-31.

GELARDI M, FIORELLA ML, TARASCO E, PASSALACQUA G, PORCELLI F. Blowing a nose black and blue. Lancet 2009 Feb 28; 373(9665): 780.

GELARDI M, RUSSO C, FIORELLA ML, FIORELLA R, CANONICA GW, PASSALACQUA G. When allergic rhinitis is not only allergic. Am J Rhinol Allergy 2009 May-Jun; 23(3): 312-5.

GELARDI M, MEZZOLI A, FIORELLA ML, CARBONARA M, DI GIOACCHINO M, CIPRANDI G. Nasal irrigation with lavonase as ancillary treatment of acute rhinosinusitis: a pilot study. J Biol Regul Homeost Agents 2009 Apr-Jun; 23(2): 79-84.

GELARDI M, FIORELLA R, FIORELLA ML, RUSSO C, SOLETI P, CIPRANDI G. Nasal-sinus polyposis: clinical-cytological grading and prognostic index of relapse. J Biol Regul Homeost Agents 2009 Jul-Sep; 23(3): 181-8.

GELARDI M, FIORELLA ML, RUSSO C, FIORELLA R, CIPRANDI G. Role of nasal cytology. Int J Immunopathol Pharmacol. 2010 Jan-Mar; 23(1 Suppl): 45-9.

GELARDI M, SPADAVECCHIA L, FANELLI P, FIORELLA ML, RUSSO C, FIORELLA R, ARMENIO L, PASSALACQUA G. Nasal inflammation in vernal keratoconjunctivitis. J Allergy Clin Immunol. 2010 Feb; 125(2): 496-8.

GELARDI M, RUSSO C, FIORELLA ML, FIORELLA R, CIPRANDI G. Inflammatory cell types in nasal polyps. Cytopathology 2010 Jun; 21(3): 201-3.

GELARDI M, VENTURA MT, FIORELLA R, FIORELLA ML, RUSSO C, CANDREVA T, CARRETTA A, PASSALACQUA G. Allergic and non-allergic rhinitis in swimmers: clinical and cytological aspects. Br J Sports Med. 2010 Jun 27.

GELARDI M, PASSALACQUA G, FIORELLA ML, MOSCA A, QUARANTA N. Nasal cytology: the "infectious spot", an expression of a morphological-chromatic biofilm. Eur J Clin Microbiol Infect Dis 2011 Sep; 30(9): 1105-9.

GELARDI M, INCORVAIA C, FIORELLA ML, PETRONE P, QUARANTA N, RUSSO C, PUCCINELLI P, ALBANI ID, RIARIO-SFORZA GG, CATTANEO E, PASSALACQUA G, FRATI F. The clinical stage of allergic rhinitis is correlated to inflammation as detected by nasal cytology. Inflamm Allergy Drug Targets 2011 Dec 1; 10(6): 472-6.

GELARDI M, INCORVAIA C, PASSALACQUA G, QUARANTA N, FRATI F. The classification of allergic rhinitis and its cytological correlate. Allergy 2011 Dec; 66(12): 1624-5.

GŁOWACKI R, STREK P, ZAGÓRSKA-SWIEZY K, SKŁADZIEŃ J, OLEŚ K, HYDZIK-SOBOCIŃSKA K, MIODOŃSKI A. Biofilm from patients with chronic rhinosinusitis. Morphological SEM studies Otolaryngol Pol. 2008; 62(3): 305-10.

GLUCK U, GEBBERS JO. Cytopathology of the nasal mucosa in smokers: a possible biomarker of air pollution? Am J Rhinol 1996; 10: 55-7.

GOLLASH A. Zur des asthmatischen sputums. Fortschritte der Medizin. 1889; 7: 361-5.

HANSEL F.K. Observation on the cytology of the secretions in allergy of the nose and paranasal sinuses. J Allergy 1934; 5: 357-66.

HEINO M. Morphological changes related to ciliogenesis in the bronchial epithelium in experimental conditions and clinical course of disease. Eur Respir J 1987; 71: S3-S39.

HOLM AF, FOKKEENS WJ. Topical corticosteroids in allergic rhinitis; effects on nasal inflammatory nasal mucosa. Clin Exsp Allergy 2001 Apr; 31(4): 529-35.

HOWART PH. Allergic Rhinitis: A rational choice of treatment. Respir Med 1989; 83: 179-88.

HOYLE BD, COSTERTON JW. Bacterial resistance to antibiotics: the role of biofilms. Prog Drug Res. 1991; 37: 91-105.

JACOBS RL, FREEDMAN PM, BOSWELL RN. Nonallergic rhinitis with eosinophils (NARES syndrome). J Allergy Clin Immunol 1981; 67: 253-62.

JACOBSON MR, JULIUSSON S, LOWHAGEN O, BALDER B, KAY AB, DURHAM SR. Effect of topical corticosteroids on seasonal increases in epithelial eosinophils and mast cells in allergic rhinitis: a comparison of nasal brush and biopsy methods. Clin Exp Allergy 1999; 29(10): 1347-55.

JETTEN AM. Growth and differentiation factors in tracheobronchial epithelium. Am J Physiol 1991; 260: L361-L373.

JOHNSTON WW. Pleural fluid. Diagnostic Cytology Seminar Acta Cytol, 23rd Annual Scientific Meeting. 1976; 20: 428-43.

JOHNSTON WW, ELSON CE. Respiratory Tract. Comprehensive Cytopathology. M. Bibbo (ed). Philadelphia: WB Saunders Company, 1991.

JOHNSTON WW, FRABLE WJ. Diagnostic Respiratory Cytopathology. Paris: Masson, 1979.

KARLSSON G, PIPKOM U. Natural allergen exposure does not influence the density of goblet cells in the mucosa of patients with seasonal allergic rhinitis. J Otorhinolaryngol 1989; 51: 171-4.

KNANI J, CAMPBELL A, ENANDER I, PETERSON CG, MICHEL FB, BOUSQUET J. Indirect evidence of nasal inflammation assessed by titration of inflammatory mediators and enumeration of cells in nasal secretions of patients with chronic rhinitis. J Allergy Clin Immunol 1992; 90: 880-9.

LAMB D, REID L. Mitotic rates, goblet cell increase and histochemical changes in mucus in rat bronchial epithelium during exposure to sulphur dioxide. J Pathol Bacteriol 1968; 96: 97-111.

LANS DM, ALFANO N, ROCKLIN R. Nasal eosinophilia in allergic and non-allergic rhinitis: Usefulness of the nasal smear in the diagnosis of allergic rhinitis. Allergy Proc 1989; 10: 275-80.

LEE HS, MAJIMA Y, SAKAKURA Y, SHINOGI J, KIM BW, KAWAGUCHI S. Quantitative cytology of nasal secretions under various conditions. Laryngoscope 1993; 103: 533-7.

LEIGH M. W., KYLANDER J.E., YANKASKAS J. R., BOUCHER R.C., 1995, "Cell proliferation in bronchial epithelium and submucosal glands of cystic fibrosis patients", in Am J Respir Cell Mol Biol, pp. 605-612.

LIPWORTH BJ, WHITE PS. Allergic inflammation in the unified airway start with the nose. Thorax 2000; 55(10): 878-81.

MALMBERG H. Symptoms of chronic and allergic rhinitis and occurrence of nasal secretion granulocytes in university students, school children and infants. Allergy 1979; 34: 389-94.

MALMBERG H, HOLOPAINEN E. Nasal smear as a screening test for immediate-type nasal allergy. Allergy 1979; 34: 331-7.

MARTUZZI M, DALLA PICCOLA B. Citologia Diagnostica e Citogenetica. Firenze: USES Edizioni Scientifiche, 1990.

MCKEE GT. Cytopathology. Mosby Wolfe, 1997.

MELTZER EO, JALOWAYSKI AA. Nasal cytology in clinical practice. Am J Rhinol 1988; 2: 47-54.

MELTZER EO, ORGEL HA, JALOWAYSKI A. Nasal Cytology. In Naclerio R. e coll., Rhinitis, Cap. 11, 175-202. New York: Marcel Dekker Inc., 1999.

MELTZER EO, ORGEL HA, ROGENES PR, FIELD EA. Nasal cytology in patients with allergic rhinitis: effects of intranasal fluticasone propionate. J Allergy Clin Immunol 1994; 94(4): 708-15.

MIDDLETON E, ELLIS E, YUNGINGER JW, REED CE, ADKINSON NF, BUSSE WW. Allergy - Principles & Pratice. Mosby Wolf, 1998.

MINIELLO OG. Colposcopy and Phase Contrast Microscopy,. Roma: CIC Edizioni Internazionali, 1998.

MONESI V. Istologia. Padova: Piccin Editore, 1976.

MYGIND N, DURHAM SR, NACLERIO RM. Plans for the management of rhinitis. In Rhinitis: mechanism and management, Ed. Naclerio Dhuram Mygind. New York: Marcel Dekker, Inc., 369-81, 1999.

MYGIND N, PEDERSEN M, NIELSEN M. Morphology of the upper airway epithelium. In Proctor DF, Andersen J (eds.). The Nose. Amsterdam: Elsevier Biomedical Press, 1982.

NICOLETTI G, MAR NICOLOSI V. Dizionario di Batteriologia Umana normale e Patologica. Salerno: Momento Medico, 1998.

OHTSUKA H, OKUDA M. Important factors in the nasal manifestations of allergy. Arch Otorhinolaryngol 1981; 233: 227-35.

OKUDA M, YEN CH, OHKUBO K, FOOANANT S, IKEDA M, PAWANKAR R. Intraepithelial cell population in the allergic nasal mucosa. Am J Rhinol 1991; 5: 219-25.

ORELL SR et al. Manual and Atlas of fine needle aspiration cytology. London: Churchill Livingston, 1992.

ORGEL HA, MELTZER EO, KEMP JP, OSTROM NK, WELCH MJ. Comparison of intranasal cromolyn sodium 4%, and oral terfenadine for allergic rhinitis: symptoms, nasal cytology, nasal ciliary clearance, and rhinomanometry. Ann Allergy 1991; 66(3): 237-44.

PALMER RJ JR, STERNBERG C. Modern microscopy in biofilm research: confocal microscopy and other approaches. Curr Opin Biotechnol. 1999; 10(3): 263-8.

PASSÀLI D. La rinite allergica: Problemi clinici e diagnostici. In Zanussi C. Trattato Italiano di Allergologia, Vol. 1, 491-506. Pavia: Selecta Medica, 1991.

PASSÀLI D. Around the nose, Editor Desiderio Passàli. Cadenzano, Firenze: Conti Tipocolor, 1988.

PELIKAN Z, PELIKAN-FILIPEK M. Cytologic changes in the nasal secretions during the immediate nasal response. J Allergy Clin Immunol 1988; 82: 1103-12.

PELIKAN Z, PELIKAN-FILIPEK M. Cytologic changes in the nasal secretions during the late nasal response. J Allergy Clin Immunol 1989; 83: 1068-79.

PELUCCHI A, CHIAPPARINO A, MASTROPASQUA B, MARAZZINI L, HERNENDEZ A, FORESI A. Effect of intranasal azelastine and beclomethasone dipropionate on nasal symptoms, nasal cytology, and bronchial responsiveness to methacholine in allergic rhinitis in response to grass pollens. J Allergy Clin Immunol 1995; Feb. (2): 515-23.

PIPKORN U, KARLSSON G. Methods for obtaining specimens from the nasal mucosa for morphological and biochemical analysis. Eur Respir J 1988; 1: 856-62.

PRINCE AS. Biofilms, antimicrobial resistance, and airway infection. N Eng J Med 2002; 347: 1110-1.

PSALTIS AJ, HA KR, BEULE AG, TAN LW, WORMALD PJ. Confocal scanning laser microscopy evidence of biofilms in patients with chronic rhinosinusitis. Laryngoscope. 2007; 117(7): 1302-6.

RICCA V, FERRERO P, BAIRO A, ROBBA S, MARCHELLO A. La citologia nasale nel monitoraggio terapeutico della rinite allergica. Giorn It Allergol Immunol Clin 1998; (8/1): 279-80.

RICCA V, FIORUCCI GC, CIPRANDI G, CANONICA GW. Il contributo del laboratorio nella diagnostica allergologica. Biochim. Clin Suppl 1983; 1/9: 45.

ROGERS DF. Airway goblet cells: responsive and adaptable frontline defenders. Eur Respir J 1994; 7: 1690-706.

ROTLAND J, DEWAR A, COX T, COLE P. Nasal brushing for the study of ciliary ultrastructure. J Clin Pathol 1982; 35: 357-9.

SANCLEMENT JA, WEBSTER P, THOMAS J, RAMADAN HH. Bacterial biofilms in surgical specimens of patients with chronic rhinosinusitis. Laryngoscope. 2005; 115(4): 578-82.

SANICO A, TOGIAS A. Noninfectious, nonallergic rhinitis (NINAR): considerations on possible mechanisms. Am J Rhinol. 1998; 12: 65-72.

SETTIPANE GA, KLEIN DE. Non-allergic rhinitis: demography of eosinophils in nasal smear, blood total eosinophil counts and IgE levels. Allergy Proc 1985; 6: 363-6.

TOBIN AJ, MOREL RE. Asking about Cells. Philadelphia: Harcourt Brace & Company Publishing, 1997.

VENTURA MT, GELARDI M, DI GIOIA R, BUQUICCHIO R, ACCETTURA G, TUMMOLO RA, ARSIENI A. Statistical evaluation and parameters of phlogosis in patients sensitized to cypress. J Biol Regul Homeost Agents 2007, 21: 41-8.

VLASTARAKOS PV, NIKOLOPOULOS TP, MARAGOUDAKIS P, TZAGAROULAKIS A, FEREKIDIS E Biofilms in ear, nose, and throat infections: how important are they? Laryngoscope 2007; 117(4): 668-73.

VOLGATE S, CHURCH MK. Allergy. Mosby-Gower, 1994.

WELCH MJ, MELTZER EO, KEMP JP et al. Comparison of two different techniques for obtaining specimens for nasal cytology. Nose-blowing vs. nasal mucosal scraping. J Allergy Clin Immunol 1991; 87: 144.

ZACCHEO D, CATTANEO L, GROSSI CE. Anatomia microscopica degli organi dell'uomo. Torino: UTET, 1973.

ZANUSSI C. Trattato Italiano di Allergologia. Pavia: Selecta Medica, 1983.

ZEIGER RS, SCHATZ M. Chronic rhinitis: a practical approach to diagnosis and treatment. Immun. Allergy Practice 1982; 4: 63-78; 4:108-18.

Index

Page numbers followed by the letter "f" are references to figures in the text

A

Actinomycetes, 109
Adenovirus, 57, 106-107
Allergens, 43, 45, 117, 126-128
Allergy, 35, 38, 42, 50, 96, 103, 115, 117, 122, 124, 126-128
α-adrenergic
– agents, 113
– drug, 103, 111
Allergen, 35, 125 – 127
Allergy 115, 120, 130
Alterations
– cellular, 19, 91, 97f, 99
– nuclear, 99, 107, 110
Alternaria, 109, 186f
Analysis of nasal cytogram
– quantitative, 91
– semiquantitative, 91
Antihistamines, 119-121, 125, 130
Apparatus ciliary 2, 10f, 19f-20f, 76, 91, 97, 97f, 134f, 136f, 148f-150f, 152f, 168-170f
Arneth classification, 29
Ascospore, 52
Aspergillus, 53, 53f, 109

B

Bacteria, 5f, 18, 30f, 43f-44f, 46-50, 55f-57f, 81f, 87, 89-93, 99-100, 100f, 102, 104f-105f, 106, 111, 119, 123, 128, 139f-141f, 145f-146f, 155-156f, 158f, 174 f, 180f, 184f-185f
Bacterial adhesion 5f, 140f, 170f
Basophilia, 5, 7, 42
Binucleation, 99, 147f, 149f-150f, 164f
Biopsy, 76
Blastospore, 52
Brushing, 73, 75

C

Caliciform mucous (goblet) cell *see* Cell
Candida, 109, 155f
Cell, 1-12
– basal, 15f, 24
– caliciform mucous (goblet) 15f, 20-23, 146f, 164f, 171f, 173f, 178f
– ciliated, 2f-3f, 10f, 15f, 19-20, 81f, 85f, 92f-93f, 97f, 101f, 102, 134f, 136f, 140f, 144f, 146f-150f, 152f, 177f, 171f, 173f, 177f-179f, 187f
– columnar 9f, 15
– inflammatory 27-44, 104
– striate, 12f, 15, 23, 23f, 179f
Centrioles, 2, 6-7, 8f, 10
Charcot-Leyden crystal (CLC), 33
Chorion, 25, 130
Chromatin, 3, 29, 32
– nuclear, 4f, 8f-9f, 21f-22f, 39-40, 42, 82, 178f
– margination, 99f
– nucleolus-associated, 4-5
Ciliary, apparatus *see* Apparatus ciliary
Ciliocytophthoria, 90-93, 100, 107, 135f, 176f, 181f, 187f
Cladosporium, 109
Conidiophores, 53-54
Coronavirus, 57, 106
Corticosteroids, 109, 119-121, 124, 130
Creola body, 33, 34f
Cytoplasmic
– granules, 30, 32, 107, 117f
– membrane, 51
– protrusions, 39
– vacuolization, 99, 100f

D

Degeneration, vacuolar, 139f, 166f
Degenerative processes, 97-98
Degranulation, 34, 34f, 90, 92-93, 118f, 126f
Desmosomes, 19, 24f
Destaining, 86
Differential interference contrast (DIC), 64
Diopter adjustment, 63
Disodium cromoglycate (DSCG), 120, 121f

E

Echo virus, 57
ECP *see* Eosinophilic cationic protein
Elastase, 30f
Elastasis, 31f
Endoplasmic reticulum, 4, 7
– – rough, 7, 7f, 8f
– – smooth, 7f-8f, 20, 23-24
Enzymes, 8, 10, 30, 30f, 33, 36f
– proteolytic, 8
Eosin, 32, 82-83
Eosinophil, 9f, 20f, 28f, 32-34, 39f, 115, 116f-119f, 121f, 124f, 128-129, 141f-142f, 144f, 149f, 151f, 154f, 164f, 170f, 176f-177f, 181f, 183f
Eosinophil-derived neurotoxin (EDN), 33
Eosinophilic
– cationic protein (ECP), 33, 33f
– peroxidase (EPO), 33, 33f
Epicoccum, 109
Epithelium
– pseudostratified ciliated, 16
– stratified pavimentous, 15f
– transition, 16
EPO *see* Eosinophilic peroxidase

Equipment and supplies, 81
Erythrocytes, 73
Euchromatin, 4f, 97
Exit pupil, 62, 63f
Exocytosis, 10, 21, 30, 35,
Exocytotic vesicles 30, 43f

F
Fixation, 78-79, 87
Formaldehyde, 111
Free radicals, 30, 31f, 123
Fungi, 51-56, 88f, 109
Fusarium, 109

G
Golgi apparatus 2, 6-8, 20
Grading 91, 130
Granulation, 8, 23, 29, 81, 179f
Granulocyte/es, 29-34

H
Haemophilus influenzae, 18, 47, 49
Helminthosporium, 109
Hematoxylin and eosin stain, 82, 83f
Hemidesmosomes, 24f
Herpes virus, 57, 106, 108f
Heterochromatin, 4, 4f, 97
Hyperchromia, 99
Hypha, 52, 85
– fungal, 110, 123
– septate, 51, 52f

I
IgA, 15, 21,11
IgE, 35-36, 36f
Images
– acquisition, 69
– archiving, 69-70, 92
Immersion oil, 65f-66f, 66, 91
Immunity, 39-40
Immunocomplexes, 31f
Inclusions
– intracytoplasmic, 9, 107
– intranuclear, 100
Inflammation 52, 99, 104, 106
– minimal persistent, 115, 115f, 116, 120, 127, 159f, 183f
Inflammatory
– agents, 43-57, 104, 106, 112f,
– cells, 27-44

– processes, 99, 100
Interferon (IFN), 40, 43
Interpupil distance, 63

K
Karyolysis, 97, 98f
Karyorrhexis, 97, 97f, 105f, 110
Klebsiella ozaenae, 131

L
Laminin, 19, 20f
Layer
– glandular, 25
– lymphoid, 25
– vascular, 25
Leukotrienes, 30f, 33f, 36f
Liquid fixatives, 73
Lymphocytes 3, 22f, 28f, 39-41, 102f, 117f-118f, 144f, 148f, 152f, 154f, 159f, 162f, 166 f, 168f-169f, 176f, 179f, 181f-182f
– B, 38, 40
– null, 39
– T, 39-40, 43
Lysosomes, 8, 179f

M
Macrophage, 43-44, 43f-44f, 155f, 159f, 172f, 176f, 184f
Major basic protein (MBP), 33, 34f
Mast cell, 35-38, 102f
Mastocytosis, 129f, 130, 153f, 161f, 164f, 166f
May-Grünwald-Giemsa (MGG) staining, 80, 81f
Membrane
– basale, 15, 25
– cytoplasmic, 51
– nuclear, 3-4
Metachromasia, 35, 83f
Metachromatic staining, 35f, 81
Metachronous movement, 11
Metaplasia, 112f, 157f
– muciparous, 111, 113, 113f, 187f
– platycellular, 111, 113, 114f
– squamous, 131, 131f
Microfilaments, 7, 8f, 23
Microphagia, 30
Microscope
– coverslip, 66

– exit pupil, 63f
– eyepiece, 61-62
– field diaphragm, 61, 68, 68f
– illuminator, 61, 68, 68f
– magnifying power, 64
– objective lens, 63
– resolution power, 64
– revolving power, 66
– stage, 67
– stand, 68
– substage condenser, 61, 67, 67f
– workstation, 69, 85f
Microscopic observation, 61, 84, 89-93
Microscopy
– electron, 6, 10f, 12f, 57
– light 4, 6-10, 16f, 59-70
– phase-contrast, 5f, 16f, 43f, 52, 53f, 70
Microtubules, 7, 10-11, 16, 17
Microvilli, 12, 12f, 19, 21, 23
Mitochondria, 8
Mota's basic lead acetate, 79
Mucociliary
– clearance, 18, 44, 47f, 107, 111, 112f
– transport, 18
Mycelium, filamentous, 51
Myxovirus, 57, 106

N
NARES *see* Non Allergic Rhinitis with Eosinophilic Syndrome
Nasal cavity, 14-16, 14f-15f, 25, 44, 47, 74, 131
Nasal provocation test, 35, 36f 115, 116f, 126f, 127
Nasal cytopathology, 95-110
Nasal
– lavage, 74-75, 75f
– smear, 78, 78f, 82
Neisseria, 18, 47, 50
Neutrophil, 4f, 9f, 28f, 29-31, 105f, 115f-119f, 144f, 150f, 158f, 162f, 165f, 166f, 174f, 180f, 182f
Non Allergic Rhinitis with Eosinophilic Syndrome, 32, 123-124, 124f, 158f, 183f
Nose blowing, 74, 74f

Nuclear
– alterations, 97, 107, 110f
– appendages, 29
– dyschromia, 97
– pyknosis, 4, 97, 97f
Nucleolus, 5, 105f, 162f, 184f
Nucleus, 3-5
Numerical aperture (NA), 65-66, 65f

O
Objective, 61, 64-65
–, lens
– – dry, 65f, 67
– – immersion, 65f, 66, 82
Optical physics, 61

P
Paramyxovirus, 57, 106
PAS staining, 56, 56f
Penicillium, 54, 54f, 109
Perez's coccobacillus, 131
Perinuclear halo, 107
Phagocytosis 8, 30, 31f, 43f-44f, 99, 172f
Photography, digital, 70
PLAN, 64
Plasma cell, 42, 42f, 104, 138f, 180f
Platelet-activating factor (PAF), 33f,
Polynucleation, 101, 107, 108f, 172f-173f
Polyposis nasal, 109, 124, 127-129, 129f
Polyps
– antrochoanal, 129
– nasal, 129-130
Pseudomonas, 18, 50, 50f
Pullularia, 109

R
Reovirus, 57
Ribosomes, 7, 7f-8f
Rhinitis
– allergic, 28, 31f, 34, 40, 75f, 102f, 115, 116f, 119, 119f, 121f, 126f, 135f, 138f, 143f, 145f, 149f, 152f, 154f, 157f, 159f, 164f-166f, 176f, 183f, 186f
– atrophic, 128, 131
– – bacterial, 100f, 104f-106f, 139f, 141f, 147f, 153f, 156f, 158f, 165f, 167f, 169f, 175f, 180f
– – viral, 148f
– - eosinophil, 115
– - infectious, 97, 148f
– - inflammatory, 28, 31f, 35
– - mastocytic, 148f
– - medicamentosa, 131
– - mycotic, 110f, 140f, 145f, 155f, 167f, 186f
– - neutrophil, 117, 127
– - pregnancy, 128
– - vasomotor, 115-128

S
Sampling
– sites, 77, 77f
– tecniques, 74-76
Slide
– mounting, 84, 84f,
– preparation, 84
– rack, 73, 81, 83, 84
Smears, inadequate, 87
Sporangiophore, 52
Spores, 51-52, 51f, 56f, 81f, 106f, 110f, 140f, 145-146f, 149f, 155f, 167f, 186f

Sporophore, 52
Staining methods
– Hematoxylin and eosin, 82
– May-Grünwald-Giemsa, 80-81f
– PAS, 56, 56f
– Toluidine blue, 35, 80, 82-83, 115
Staining solution, 82
Staphylococcus, 47
Stemphyllium, 109
Streptococcus, 18, 47-48, 180f
Supranuclear hyperchromatic stria (SHS), 19-20, 81, 136f, 144f, 148f-150f, 152f, 168f, 171f, 177f-178f

T
Thallus, 51
Thrush, 109
Toluidine blue *see* Staining methods
Tumor necrosis factor (TNF), 40
Tunica propria, 25, 25f

V
Vacuolar degeneration, 139f, 166f
Vacuole (s), 8, 9f, 142f, 176f, 184f
– digestive (s), 30, 43, 44f
– intracytoplasmic, 9f, 118, 152f, 173f
Virus, 57, 106-107

X
Xylol, 73, 83, 86

Y
Yeasts, 51, 109